S0-BWV-772

# THE LOSER-FRIENDLY DIET

# THE LOSER-FRIENDLY DIET

by Malcolm J. Nicholl

*M. EVANS & COMPANY, INC.*

Nicholl, Malcom J.
The loser-friendly diet / Malcolm J. Nicholl.
p. cm.
Includes bibliographical references and index
ISBN 0-87131-712-5 : $19.95
1. Reducing diets. I. Title.
RM222.2.N493 1993
613.2'–dc20 92-32952
CIP

M. Evans and Company, Inc.
216 East 49th Street
New York, New York 10017

Manufactured in the United States of America

9 8 7 6 5 4 3 2 1

# ACKNOWLEDGMENTS

I owe a debt of gratitude to the talented individuals who contributed so enthusiastically to the creation of this book: Fred Dickey, Katherine Greene, Peter Kenyon, Paul Lapolla, Susan J. Meyerott, Tara Pheneger, and Colin Rose, and my colleagues in the Uni-Vite family. I am grateful, too, for the support and encouragement of the medical experts who painstakingly reviewed the manuscript, Phyllis Crapo, R.D., Edward S. Horton, M.D., Jerrold M. Olefsky, M.D. and Jacqueline Stordy, B.Sc. Ph.D. Any errors are mine, not theirs. And a special thanks to my wife, Maggie, for understanding the "lost" evenings and weekends.

## IMPORTANT NOTICE

The recommended way to lose weight with *The Loser-Friendly Diet* is by making meal selections totaling at least 800 calories a day. Such a caloric intake makes the program fall into the category of a Low-Calorie Diet. Anyone choosing to consume fewer calories would be embarking on a Very Low-Calorie Diet and must do so only with their physician's monitoring, and for no longer than three consecutive weeks at a time. Both Very Low-Calorie Diets and Low-Calorie Diets are not appropriate for growing children, adolescents, pregnant and lactating women, and individuals with cardiac, liver, or kidney disease. A doctor's supervision is required for the elderly, and for individuals with known medical conditions such as gout, gallbladder disease, Type II diabetes, and high blood pressure.

# CONTENTS

# FOREWORD

OBESITY IS AN exceedingly common problem in the United States as well as other Western countries. In fact, in the recent Surgeon General's report, obesity was characterized as an "epidemic" and should be considered as a disorder directly linked to a country's economic prosperity, cultural mores, and food availability.

In addition to esthetic considerations, obesity is associated with a number of health risks including diabetes, heart disease, and hypertension. Consequently, the successful prevention and treatment of obesity has enormous health advantages to individuals and to society as a whole. Although these facts are generally well recognized, successful treatment of obesity remains a difficult problem.

Over the years a number of approaches to weight reduction have been proposed, ranging from total starvation to moderate caloric restriction to various "fad" diets. Generally these programs have met with mixed success at best. Recently, a great deal of attention has been focused on the Very Low-Calorie Diet (VLCD) and Low-Calorie Diet (LCD) methods of weight management.

A VLCD program usually refers to a daily caloric intake of 600 calories or less, whereas diets of 800 (or somewhat greater) calories are designated as LCDs. The basic principle underlying most VLCDs and LCDs is that specially formulated food, which provides a full day's nutritional complement of vitamins, minerals, protein, and other essential nutrients, with only a small number of calories, can be used to eliminate worry about obtaining adequate nutrition. In addition, this approach decreases the stress of making food choices.

If "empty calories" refers to soda pop, candy, and other food sources which provide calories but few nutrients, then the calories incorporated into properly formulated LCDs are indeed quite full. Many clinical studies have utilized such programs with excellent success, and this approach to weight loss has been proven to be highly effective in motivated individuals.

This book outlines the principles and provides the full details of the Loser-Friendly Diet. The Loser-Friendly Diet combines a formulated LCD program with exercise and behavior modification components in a comprehensive lifelong approach to weight management. The program is described in an easy-to-read, practical way which should appeal to a wide spectrum of potential dieters. Relevant clinical trials and other research studies are reviewed and cited, lending sound medical and scientific support to the validity and efficacy of this LCD approach. In addition, the book contains a great deal of basic nutritional information and thus, can serve as a useful resource, even to non-dieters. The book is also loaded with helpful practical suggestions for using the various food, including recipes, cooking tips, and ways to add flexibility to the diet plan. Although the general principles of the LCD approach are clearly discussed, the importance of tailoring the diet program to each person's lifestyle and needs is stressed.

Provided proper medical precautions and indications are followed, the LCD dietary approach is also quite safe. The marked calorie reduction provided by this diet leads to a rapid and satisfying rate of weight loss. This is gratifying and can be highly motivating to the dieter, providing him or her with the extra psychological boost which often means the difference between success and failure.

Please remember that this diet is not for everybody and that certain precautions are necessary. For example, pregnant women, growing children, and teenagers should not be on such diets. In addition, there are some medical conditions which preclude this dietary approach, and others in which close physician supervision is mandatory. All of these are discussed in more detail in the body of this book. As long as these guidelines are followed by dieters and their physicians, then the Loser-Friendly Diet should be both effective and safe.

Losing weight is only the first step in an overall weight-management program. As many dieters know, keeping the weight off is often the most difficult part. Many overweight individuals have successfully lost weight only to regain it and then repeat the cycle over and over again. In recent years, clinical research studies have shown that behavior modification and exercise are important components of a successful weight-maintenance phase to an overall obesity-management program.

This book provides an easy-to-read, excellent overview of a number of tactics to achieve modification of eating behavior as well as to introduce regular exercise into your daily habits. All of these procedures are designed to put control back into the dieter's hands.

Studies have shown that the overall amount of weight loss is about the same on an 800-calorie-a-day diet compared to more restricted caloric-reduction regimens. Stringent VLCD approaches offering only 30-40 grams of protein per day may represent a marginal protein intake in some individuals (e.g. heavy, active men). By allowing more calories (at least 800 Kcal/day), the Loser-Friendly Diet provides additional protein (59-81 grams/day) satisfying the protein Recommended Daily Allowance (RDA) for almost all people.

In summary this book provides a thorough description of a formulated diet-based LCD plan called the Loser-Friendly Diet. This diet plan has an excellent track record for being highly successful and well tolerated. Once weight loss is achieved, the maintenance phase begins. For long-term success diet, behavior modification, and incorporation of exercise into daily life are all important. The information provided in this book will be of great help to the overweight person attempting to construct a lifelong approach to weight management.

Jerrold M. Olefsky, M.D.
Professor of Medicine
University of California,
San Diego

Edward S. Horton, M.D.
Chairman, Department
of Medicine
University of Vermont

Phyllis Crapo, R.D.
Associate Professor
of Medicine
University of
California, San Diego

# THE LOSER-FRIENDLY DIET

# 1

# HOW IT ALL BEGAN

WELCOME TO *The Loser-Friendly Diet.* By opening this book you have taken a vital step toward achieving the size and shape that you want to be. You can do it by following this proven program for weight loss and weight maintenance—a realistic program that has already helped millions across the globe.

If you've tried everything else and failed, *The Loser-Friendly Diet* is for you. If you want to lose ten pounds, fifty pounds, one hundred pounds or even more, there's a loser-friendly plan suitable for you. Even if you don't have fat to shed, you will gain enormous benefits for yourself and your entire family because this is not just a "diet" in the sense of losing weight, it's a blueprint for healthy eating that can fit into everyone's lifestyle.

*The Loser-Friendly Diet* has evolved out of more than sixty years of scientific research, particularly in the area known to the scientific community as Very Low-Calorie Diets and Low-Calorie Diets in which typical meals are replaced with specially formulated, nutritionally fortified meals. (Scientists disagree on the difference between a Very Low-Calorie Diet (VLCD) and a Low-Calorie Diet (LCD) but, in general, under 800 calories a day is a VLCD; 800 to 1,200 calories can be classified LCD.)

*The Loser-Friendly Diet* is a low-calorie plan providing a recommended minimum of 800 calories a day. It is a program which has been promoted around the world as "The Micro Diet" and therefore, in this book, you will find many specific references to dieters' experiences with The Micro Diet.

So what is the loser-friendly Micro Diet? First, let me make it very clear:

MICRO, in this context, doesn't mean small or that the program involves microwave cooking!

DIET doesn't just mean weight loss!

The use of the word "Micro" indicates the computer-age yet "loser-friendly" sophistication of the program. In the same way that the revolutionary micro chip has miniaturized computers, food technologists have packed all of the essential nutrients (including the *micro* nutrients) into low-calorie, well-balanced meals. The word "Diet" is used in its original context—not meaning "to lose weight" but indicating, as Webster's puts it, "habitual nourishment" or "food and drink regularly provided or consumed." In other words, your daily diet.

The Micro Diet is, in fact, a comprehensive weight management system in complete accord with the key findings of the *U.S. Surgeon General's Report on Nutrition and Health*, the British Committee on Medical Aspects of Food Policy, and other leading authorities. The landmark Surgeon General's report, published in 1988, declared: "Overweight patients should be provided with counseling and assistance in the development of diets low in calories and high in essential nutrients, as well as lifestyle modifications that include high levels of physical activity to achieve appropriate weight goals."

That approach is exactly what you will find in this book, including:

- a low-calorie, low-fat, eating plan which provides complete nutrition
- lifestyle modification—for permanent success, you'll discover how to make pain-free adjustments in your habits
- exercise—a gentle step-by-step program which shows you how getting fit can be fun and
- personal support—you choose the kind of help you want from a diet "advisor" who helps you on a one-to-one basis or at motivating group sessions.

*The Loser-Friendly Diet* is a program which:

- produces meaningful and motivational weight loss.
- harnesses the latest in food technology to create delicious, nutritious, convenient, quick-fix meals.
- is extremely flexible, letting you lose at the rate you want by offering a variety of choices.
- is safe—extensive clinical testing lies behind the concept upon which the program is based.
- makes economic sense, being within the reach of everyone's pocketbook.
- and introduces a new, enjoyable lifestyle to enable you to stay slim and trim.

It is perfect for the fast-paced demands of today's society.

## *IN THE BEGINNING*

By profession, for many years I was a journalist—not a scientist, physician, or dietitian—and this has given me a tremendous advantage in my investigation of weight management programs. For, as a journalist, I was trained to be skeptical and schooled in the art of asking penetrating questions. I originally approached the subject of dieting, therefore, with a healthy degree of cynicism, subscribing to the belief that "diets don't work," and when I came across the concept upon which The Mico Diet is based I found it hard to swallow, even though the report was published in *The Lancet,* an internationally respected medical journal. The scientific evidence seemed beyond reproach, but firmly entrenched in my mind was that traditional dietary myth: the body needs at least 1,000–1,500 calories a day.

However, I began to investigate further. I interviewed eminent researchers at universities and hospitals throughout Europe and the U.S. I delved into the historical development of very low-calorie and low-calorie diets, reading medical papers reporting on clinical trials of thousands of volunteers. Above all, I spoke with scores of the early "guinea pigs." Time and again, these people told the same story: They had lost weight rapidly (some of them for the first time in their lives), they felt well and energetic, and most important, they had managed to keep the weight off.

Many had even successfully and safely used nutritionally complete diets containing as few as 330 calories a day. Scientists had made the point that it was not the calories that counted, it was the nutritional quality of those calories. Over a period of months my initial cynicism gave way to a conviction that, finally, a real solution to the desperate problem of obesity had been found.

Quite independently, British entrepreneur Peter Kenyon had come across the same concept, reached the same conclusion and determined that it was time the overweight British public was given the opportunity to benefit from this weight control breakthrough. A personal weight problem was also a powerful motivator. After years of vigorous exercise playing rugby, he had settled into a fairly sedentary existence, which, in turn, had led to a typical middle-aged spread.

Together with fellow entrepreneurs Colin Rose and Joanna Downs, Peter approached one of Britain's leading manufacturers of nutritional food for hospitals and gave them the task of formulating "the best low-calorie, nutritionally complete diet... meals containing the ideal balance of all of the essential nutrients." Clinical trials were then arranged at the University of Surrey's Department of Biochemistry. The results were a complete success, impressing the experienced team of doctors and nutritionists involved. Peter, himself, lost fourteen pounds in twenty-eight days.

I was impressed, too, and decided to move from the United States, where I was living at the time, back to Great Britain to help launch the program to the British public. I found that largely through word-of-mouth recommendation, hundreds of people had already started the diet, many in the Guildford area where the University of Surrey is situated. By September 1983 about 1,000 people were following the diet and experiencing remarkable results. Word of their success spread quickly and suddenly thousands more were clamoring for The Micro Diet. A company called Uni-Vite Nutrition was formed to cope with the ever-increasing demand.

Through advertising in prestigious medical journals we brought the weight-loss plan to the attention of health professionals. Many tried the program for themselves, and soon doctors, nurses, and even skeptical dietitians—when they saw the results—began recommending it. We threw ourselves wholeheartedly into the project. Our goal: "to improve the health and quality of life of all the peoples of this planet." It was a heartfelt, if somewhat ambitious, corporate mission. And then it started to become reality. Within three years The Micro Diet was a well-known name in Great Britain and the Uni-Vite Corporation's growth was being hailed by *The Times* of London as "the sort of success usually associated with high technology breakthroughs." The program has since expanded throughout the world as people of other countries have sought to achieve the same benefits, and the term "micro diet" has entered the language (even in scientific journals) as a generic description for nutritionally complete, low-calorie diets in the same manner that people commonly refer to "Xeroxing" when they mean photocopying.

The stunning success of The Micro Diet has been exciting and challenging. But what is even more rewarding is the very real impact on people's lives. We have received literally thousands of letters and calls from triumphant dieters, delighted to have finally conquered their overweight problem. Many have commented on an overall improvement in their health.

The real-life results really do speak for themselves. Ask Mandy Shires, Miss United Kingdom of 1985, and runner-up in the Miss World event, who could not have won the coveted titles without losing twenty-eight pounds. Or Patti Carlson, of Bloomingdale, Illinois, who in 1988 became the first American "Micro Dieter of the Year" by getting rid of more than 100 pounds—and has kept it off. Or *Lifestyles of the Rich and Famous* star, Robin Leach, who lost twenty-eight pounds and says, "If I can lose weight with my way of life, anyone can."

You could also ask any of the tens of thousands of Micro Diet "Advisors." These are people who have been so impressed with their own experience that they, in turn, have made the commitment to help others by sharing the benefits of The Micro Diet by becoming distributors in their local community. It is the Advisors who provide the support and encouragement that every dieter realistically needs to achieve his or her goal. They are a vital element in our full-spectrum program and they are located in thousands of towns and neighborhoods throughout the U.S., Canada, Great Britain, and more than thirty other countries.

Since the summer of 1987, Peter Kenyon and myself, aided by a nationwide network of Advisors, have taken on the challenge of helping the country with the worst obesity problem of all—the United States. Our success here is proving to be just as sensational as in Great Britain where the country's biggest-selling daily newspaper, *The Sun*, heralded the program with the headline "Make the flab vanish with Micro Magic." A regional newspaper,

*The Darlington Evening Dispatch*, came out with the equally exuberant proclamation, "The Miracle Micro Diet," while articles such as "Micro Diet aids inch war" and "New way to beat the bulge" have been commonplace. The program has cut across all sections of society. World-class beauty queens, elite athletes, Malaysian sultans, TV and movie stars, international politicians, and even (according to one newspaper) British royalty, have all discovered the benefits of this remarkable system.

In this book, I provide the full background to the development of low-calore dieting in general, and The Micro Diet, specifically, and I bring you up-to-date with the very latest published and *unpublished* scientific research. You will read what it's like to go on the diet, and you'll discover how to improve your short-term and long-term success. You'll be impressed and motivated by the stories of dieters who have successfully travelled down the same road before you, people whose lives have been transformed. *Real people. Real names.*

I have tried to ensure that this book answers all of the questions that you, your doctor, or dietitian may want to raise. I make no apology for the enthusiasm with which it is written. Over the last few years I have met so many successful Micro Dieters whose newfound enthusiasm for life is infectious, people who have lost fifty, one hundred, one hundred fifty pounds, and more. When you hear first-hand the dramatic benefits they have experienced, when you are told countless times, "The Micro Diet has changed my life," it is hard not to share that enthusiasm. My skepticism was overcome a long time ago and today I am no longer a journalist but proud to be chairman of the company behind The Micro Diet. For millions of people, being overweight is a serious, worrying, and depressing problem, and I am grateful to be involved in a genuine breakthrough that makes a solution so readily available. I am delighted to be able to share with you a diet that *does* work.

## ■ A CASE STUDY

### LINDA GUILL: SUICIDE WITH A KNIFE AND FORK

Linda Guill weighed 276 pounds and spent her days slumped in a recliner, "eating, dozing, hurting, crying, and eating some more. I was committing suicide with a knife and fork," she says.

Doctor after doctor had already warned her that if she did not make some serious changes in her eating habits, there was a good chance she would not live to pick up Social Security. "One doctor finally lost his temper and told me that if I didn't lose weight I might not be around next year. I was a very sick and unhappy person. I had tried every diet you have ever heard about. The results were always the same. I would lose some weight and then regain it and more when stress hit my life. I could not shop. I could not do housework. I even had difficulty walking from my recliner to the car because of chest pain.

"Every time I looked in the mirror I saw this huge, gigantic monster looking back at me with dead eyes. I was actually living in a flesh-and-blood prison convinced there was no way out. I remember standing in a grocery store checkout line and a little boy asking me if I was going to have twins or triplets. I wanted to die. Everyone around me knew I wasn't pregnant."

Linda, thirty-nine years old, and five foot, four inches tall, was scared to sleep at night for fear she wouldn't wake up. "The nights were terrifying. I was afraid I was going to smother in my own fat. I would lie on my side and put pillows under my stomach to try and hold it out level so I could breathe. I would go to sleep and wake up after fifteen to twenty minutes with a crushing pain in my chest, gasping for breath."

Her worst moment came one day when, sitting in her recliner in her Odessa, Texas, home, she suffered agonizing chest pains. "I thought I was having a heart attack. The emergency services were called and I remember sitting there listening to the screeching sound of the siren." The house and yard filled up with friends and neighbors, she says, "and instead of worrying about dying I was terrified that the paramedics would not be able to lift me into the ambulance."

Fortunately, what Linda experienced was not a heart attack but a similar chest pain due to her rheumatism. The scare, however, was enough to convince her that something had to be done about her weight problem. She went on The Micro Diet and lost eight-and-a-half pounds the first week, twenty-nine pounds the first month and forty-seven pounds during the first three months. She went on to get rid of 109 pounds in a year and five months, lost nineteen inches from her waist and fourteen inches from her hips.

"What is amazing to me," says Linda, "is that I lost the first seventy pounds sitting in my recliner and the next twenty without an exercise program, just being more active in my day-to-day chores. Now that I have finally added a mild exercise program of walking my dogs and swimming, I'm firming up, and feeling better than ever."

Today, her life has completely turned around. "The Micro Diet saved my life and it changed my life. You can't imagine the joy of being able to bend over and pick something up off the floor; the thrill of walking through a shopping mall and passing others because I can walk so fast. Instead of living with constant ulcer pain, if I have a pain in my stomach now I wonder what it is. I go to bed at night, tired from a full day's work, instantly drop off to a sound sleep and then wake up refreshed before the alarm goes off. It's an unbelievable joy. My days are filled with encouraging others to lose their excess weight, walking, yard work, housework, laughing—everything but sitting in a recliner. I now live life filled with the pleasures of a healthy body."

Linda unashamedly admits that she used to describe herself as "the fattest fat person that ever lived." She says, "I was two hundred seventy-six pounds of fat hanging on a bone structure that was screaming for help. My friend, The Micro Diet, with its delicious food has taken over one hundred pounds off of me. It has also given me muscle tone, flexibility, and a joy for life I have not known in over twenty-five years and it also helps me maintain my weight loss. My other friend is my Advisor, Sal Serio, and he's lost over ninety pounds himself. Three years after losing my excess weight he still continues to call me at least once or twice a month. If I call him he always calls me back in fifteen to twenty minutes. I've always felt he was there for me. He's like a big brother to me. Just knowing he's there for support helps.

# 2

# THE WIN-WIN WEIGH TO GO

IN THE 17TH CENTURY, the fleshy nudes of Rubens were portrayed as the ideal of female beauty. Even up until this century in many Western countries moderate obesity was considered a sign of health. In fact, poverty and malnutrition were so prevalent that a corpulent body was a status symbol, a sign of social and financial well-being. But today, modern society favors a slim physique. Just look around you—magazine advertisements, TV commercials, billboards—and you'll find that all of the "beautiful people," obviously living the good life, are slim and healthy looking.

The overweight person, whenever his or her existence is acknowledged, is either the comedian, the butt of someone else's humor, or is portrayed as stupid, lazy, or ineffectual. Discrimination against the overweight person is rampant. One study revealed that 16% of employers candidly said that they would not hire overweight women under any circumstances; another 44% reported they would not hire them in certain situations. Overweight executives, it was discovered, are generally paid less. Even a group of seventy-seven physicians unsympathetically characterized their obese patients as "weak-willed, ugly, and awkward."

"Fat discrimination" is such a hot topic that countless radio and television talk shows have addressed the issue. Sally Jessy Raphael, for instance, devoted an entire program to the subject and gave the stage to an overweight woman who had been barred from boarding an airplane until she bought an extra ticket, a girl who claimed she had been rejected from the high school cheerleading squad because of her size, and a male business executive who found that after buying breakfast at McDonald's there was nowhere for him to sit—he couldn't squeeze into the fixed seating arrangement.

Pattie Petko, of Slatington, Pennsylvania, can certainly empathize with Sally Jessy's guests as she has run the entire gamut of discriminatory experiences when applying for jobs, out shopping, at work, and even at home. Pattie, who at age 39 had reached the weight of 268 pounds, tells how she was once rejected for a front office secretarial post. Although she was a college graduate, the job went instead to a high school graduate. The employer's reason: She might not fit in and might be ridiculed because of her size.

Says Pattie, "Some employers regard overweight people as being substandard and less than proficient in their job capabilities. It's amazing that you'll find people being hired, not for their qualifications, but because they personify what is desired by the public from an appearance point of view."

Even when she did get a job, the insults did not stop. Pattie recalls the day her boss was taking her out for lunch and joked about needing to take out a loan. On another occasion she climbed onto a desk to change a light bulb only to hear him make a derisive remark about the possibility of the desk collapsing. Shopping in a petite woman's store for her niece, the salesperson repeatedly and rudely told her "we don't carry *your* size"—until Pattie stormed out. At home, she grew up being called "fatty Pattie," and her father, she says, would berate her for eating dessert, and once told her that because of her weight he hated to tell people she was his daughter.

Says Pattie, "I'd heard so many insults over the years from so many people that I got to be pretty thick-skinned. But overweight people know they are overweight. They don't need to be reminded all the time. No matter what size a person is, or what a person looks like, we all deserve to be treated with the utmost dignity and respect."

During more than twenty years of dieting, Pattie says she tried virtually everything from the grapefruit diet, to the hot dog diet, to organized slimming classes. She would often lose some weight, only to watch with horror as it came piling back on. Then she discovered The Micro Diet, and in under seven months lost ninety-five pounds and forty-seven inches just in time to achieve her goal: celebrating her fortieth birthday with an hourglass figure.

"I have been able to achieve something I never thought possible. Not only do I have a waistline, but Good Lord, I can actually see my toes," says Pattie who went on to lose a total of 105 pounds, which she has maintained for more than a year.

As a casting director in the glamorous world of Hollywood, 230-pound Susan Henderson found that daily contact with what she calls "the pretty people" was an ugly situation.

"Being fat was not only a humbling experience, but an educational one as well," says Susan, who rapidly gained eighty pounds after being prescribed heavy doses of cortisone. "I had never had a weight problem before. I had been able to eat anything I wanted without gaining extra pounds, so becoming fat was an awful experience. I learned to my disgust that fat people are treated like second-class citizens. People seem to think that you have no self-control, or will-power, and you're treated like dirt."

Sometimes you're also treated as if you don't even exist, says Susan, who vividly recalls one of the most embarrassing experiences of her life—being trapped in an elevator. "I was stuck for over an hour with a guy straight out of *GQ;* you know the kind—they think every moment is a Kodak moment. Well, he never spoke to me the whole time. I can practically guarantee you that I would have had some attention if I hadn't been so overweight. When I got out of that elevator, I looked up to Heaven and said, 'OK, God, I'm humble, now make me thin.'"

Susan is now a shadow of her former self, having lost eighty pounds and kept it off for at least a year.

Legal secretary Doreen Davis of Mesa, Arizona, also knows the pain of discrimination. "I was ridiculed and scorned for years," she says. "My children were ashamed of me and did not want me to attend their school affairs. They even went so far as to not bring home the announcements of back-to-school functions because they did not want their teachers to see me. At social events, I was ostracized and ignored.

"An employment counselor once told me that I was unemployable at any 'decent' job because I was too fat, even though I held a college degree and had many skills. The men I wanted to date after my divorce did not want anything to do with me, and many of them made cruel and cutting remarks regarding my being fat.

I was accused of 'allowing myself to get that way' and 'wanting to be that way.' Nothing could have been further from the truth."

Five-foot-three, 235 pound Doreen, who attributes her weight gain to a combination of having four children and hormone medication, was always looking for an escape from an overweight body. Her dieting history is a veritable "who's who" of the weight-loss industry, including, unfortunately, just about every fad diet foisted on a public desperate for "the solution."

Says Doreen, "On all of those other diets, I never lost more than five or ten pounds. With The Micro Diet I lost seventy-five pounds in seven months and I've maintained that for a year. My blood pressure has dropped from one-fifty over ninety-four to one hundred and five over eighty. My cholesterol and triglycerides have also dramatically dropped. There isn't a day goes by that people don't compliment me. It's so much fun to go into a clothing store and have a choice. I love life again."

Pattie, Susan, and Doreen are representative of the pain suffered by the overweight person in a society which reveres sports stars and fashion models. And they are by no means alone. The extent of the torment is clearly revealed in surveys of severely overweight people. In one fascinating survey conducted by the University of Florida's Department of Psychiatry, researchers questioned forty-seven former overweight people who had maintained a 100-pound weight loss for three years. When given hypothetical choices, they said they would prefer being deaf, dyslexic, diabetic, or having heart disease to being overweight again. Leg amputation was preferred by 91.5%, and legal blindness by 89.4%. (One subject was quoted as saying, "When you're blind, people want to help you. No one wants to help you when you're fat.") Given the choice of being normal weight or a severely obese multimillionaire, ALL of them chose to be slim.

"These findings provide eloquent testimony to the pain of obesity; they call for ever more compassion and empathy on the part of those of us who treat obese persons," commented leading researchers Albert J. Stunkard and Thomas A. Wadden, of the University of Pennsylvania's Department of Psychiatry.

## *DO YOU REALLY NEED TO LOSE WEIGHT?*

A survey conducted in 1992 by the Gallup Poll showed that the average American woman is 5 foot, 4 inches tall and weighs

142 pounds, but she'd like to be 5-foot-6 inches, and weigh 129 pounds. The average man is 5 foot, 10 inches and weighs 180 pounds. He'd like to be 5-foot-11 inches and 171 pounds. That partly explains why every year fifty million Americans go on a diet. But do they all *really need* to lose weight? For many people the desire to look good, or avoid the pain of discrimination may be valid enough reasons. But let's put the pressures of society to one side. There's a far more important, motivating factor, and that's your health. Quite simply, the more overweight you become, the greater the health risks.

Obesity is a killer; it causes or contributes to an array of life-threatening ailments such as heart disease, high blood pressure, diabetes mellitus, kidney disease, gall bladder disease, and some forms of cancer. In spite of the ever-increasing wealth of information and a constant barrage of publicity, health educators have been fighting a losing battle, and the problem is actually getting worse. The American population as a whole is becoming *more* overweight.

According to the *Surgeon General's Report on Nutrition and Health*, issued during the tenure of C. Everett Koop, obesity affects about thirty-four million Americans between the ages of twenty to seventy-four, with the poor and minorities being afflicted the most. Just think about it: More than one of every four adults is overweight. Worst of all—middle-aged black women. A staggering 45% of them are classed as overweight.

And it is now widely acknowledged that even "mild" obesity is a cause for concern, especially if you have a family history of heart disease and diabetes, or have already developed high blood pressure. A Harvard Medical School study published in 1990, reviewing the medical history of over 100,000 women, discovered that even mild-to-moderate obesity substantially increased the risk of coronary disease in middle-aged women:

FACT: The risk of developing high blood pressure is up to 5.6 times greater if you are obese.

FACT: There is a three to four times greater likelihood of developing gallstones.

FACT: The chances of becoming diabetic are three times greater.

FACT: There is double the possibility of having high cholesterol.

Moreover, it is a biological fact that women tend to store fat in their thighs and buttocks, creating "pear shape" obesity; men tend to store fat in their abdomens, the "potbelly" or "apple shape" obesity we see every day. It has now become clear that apple shape obesity substantially increases the risk of a stroke or heart disease. Men whose waists are bigger than their hips fall into the risk category, as do women whose waist measurement is more than 80% of their hip size.

Another Harvard study, published in 1992, conservatively estimated the annual economic consequences of obesity in the United States (health care costs combined with lost work hours) at $39.3 billion.

## *THE WEIGHT-LOSS TREADMILL*

Let's be honest. With most diet programs, fewer than 5% of people who actually manage to lose their excess weight are able to keep it off in the long term. The well-known "yo-yo" syndrome (losing weight and regaining it) is borne out by the depressing statistic that many dieters embark on as many as fourteen different diets in a lifetime. One survey of dieters, in fact, discovered that 95% of them had dieted before and failed.

Dieters often reveal years of agony on a weight-loss treadmill. I've lost count of meetings where many depressed, overweight women such as Pattie, Susan, and Doreen (and men, too) will stand up to confess "I've tried everything!" and then back up that statement with a list of failures: calorie-counting, high-protein diets, high-carbohydrate diets, high-fiber diets, the grapefruit diet, the beer drinker's diet, or, quite often, one of those contrived diets named after some exotic location such as Beverly Hills or Hawaii. The list is endless.

Failed dieters have told me about attending weekly weight-loss clubs for months, or they will have been to the doctor for diuretics, or, believe it or not, to be injected with the urine of pregnant women! Alternatively, they will have spent a fortune at a commercial diet center or hospital clinic. Some will have turned to acupuncture, hypnosis, or starvation. Others will have resorted to one of the seemingly obvious quack diets. You know the ones—the pill which makes you lose weight while you sleep. Dream on! Or the diet patch which you apply to your wrist to curb your appetite. Frankly, you'd be better off sticking it over your mouth!

Beware, too, of the "starch blockers," the "fat blockers," the "fat magnets," and the ads which say, "We will pay you $1,000 to lose weight," or "Eat all you want and still lose weight." If it sounds too good to be true, it usually is. There is no "magic bullet." Morbidly obese individuals have even entered hospitals for surgery such as intestinal bypass and stomach stapling, while others have had liposuction, or their jaws wired.

Carolyn Hester has tried them all—the fad diets, the commercial weight-loss centers, the supermarket products, and even stomach stapling. Nothing compares, she says, with The Micro Diet.

"I want the whole world to know that they can lose weight, thanks to The Micro Diet. It has filled me with energy and life," says the forty-three-year-old mother of five (and grandmother of two), who so far has lost ninety pounds. "I couldn't even enjoy my granddaughters, and now I can play on the floor with them, go swimming, and walking with them. The Micro Diet has made me feel so much better about myself. For the first time in my life I know I will make it and keep the weight off. The Micro Diet works with your lifestyle. So many people are scared of diets because they change their lifestyle. The Micro Diet makes it easy."

Carolyn, of Ardmore, Oklahoma, weighed 262 pounds when she started The Micro Diet. She is down to 172, working on losing another seventy pounds, and in no hurry. "I won't lose it overnight, but I didn't gain it overnight, either. The great thing is that I feel I am turning from a caterpillar into a beautiful butterfly, day by day. I couldn't walk through my house without huffing and puffing. Now I can run up and down the stairs with a smile on my face."

Carolyn's weight problems began a little over ten years ago when, at about the same time, she stopped smoking, and had a hysterectomy. What happened with the other diets she tried? With one diet, she found that the meals were difficult to prepare because of special ingredients that were required. "I was always going to the store to buy something." Through a commercial weight-loss center she lost five pounds a month. The meals, she says, tasted good but she was always hungry, and thought the program too expensive. As a last resort she turned to stomach stapling. The night before the first scheduled procedure she got cold feet and backed out, but had it performed seven months later. She spent two weeks in the hospital on liquids only and after going home another two weeks on liquids. It cost thousands of dollars.

She did lose forty pounds, but feels it wasn't worth it. "I felt horrible. I was irritable and had no energy. I was still hungry. I craved food and I couldn't eat. I could only take about three tablespoons of food a day. If I had one bite more I would be in terrible pain. There were days when I would just cry. I felt weak and nervous. I wouldn't recommend it to anyone. Why should anyone go through that kind of pain when The Micro Diet is available?" Why indeed?

## *THE MYTH OF THE YO-YO*

So what is the point of going on yet another diet? You've been on five diets already, lost weight, regained it—and added a few extra pounds each time. It's a sad and all too familiar story. Many experts have argued that "yo-yo dieting" or "weight cycling" increases cardiovascular risk, such as cholesterol and blood pressure. Repeated efforts at dieting have also been said to create a decrease in your resting metabolic rate (the rate at which your body burns calories). The end result: They claim it becomes harder and harder to lose weight with each fresh attempt. Indeed, some studies with rats and college-age wrestlers with a history of yo-yo dieting have seemed to validate this theory.

But take heart.

The very latest research shows that the failed dieter should never give up hope because there are no significant health hazards associated with yo-yo dieting and your body's metabolic rate does not permanently change.

Researchers in Cambridge, England, addressed the issue in a number of highly creative ways by looking at involuntary weight cycling in women living in a remote African village, by establishing an eighteen-week study of moderately obese British women, and through analyzing the results of experiments with small animals subjected to bouts of weight loss and weight gain.

Their conclusion as published in 1992 in *The American Journal of Clinical Nutrition:* "Weight cycling is not associated with harmful effects to body composition."

The researchers from the prestigious Dunn Clinical Nutrition Centre in Cambridge studied women of child-bearing age in a village in The Gambia. For about forty years the villagers have suffered through an annual "hungry season" which occurs when the previous year's food supplies have started to run out and before the current year's harvest. The average weight loss each year during the period of starvation was about thirteen pounds, with most women cycling 50% to 60% of their fat stores each year. The Gambian women who also undergo constantly repeated cycles of pregnancy and lactation have to endure harsh nutritional conditions with a diet low in high-quality protein. But in spite of these facts, to their astonishment the researchers found that the Africans lost less lean body mass than women they studied in Britain who were on a diet but had not repeatedly tried to lose weight.

The researchers' conclusion was that the African women were perfect examples of the human ability to physically adapt to periods of feast and famine. And they went even further. They commented: "Because an abundant and reliable food supply in Western society is a very recent phenomenon on an evolutionary time-scale, it seems logical that modern man should still possess this ability, and that weight cycling should therefore be benign."

In other words, no problem.

In the British experiment, eleven women volunteers were studied for eighteen weeks and put through three cycles of two weeks of dieting followed by four weeks of eating whatever they wished. During the three diet periods, the patients consumed 445 calories a day, and average weight loss was 9.75 pounds, followed by 7.25 pounds in the second cycle, and during the third period, 6.55 pounds. Average total weight loss at the end of the eighteen weeks, because of weight gain during the "free-eating"periods, was only thirteen pounds. Significantly, however, there was no decrease in the basal metabolic rate and no detrimental impact on the amount of lean body mass lost versus pure fat loss.

The researchers commented: "These results refute the assertion that the decrease in metabolic rate associated with dieting, even on several occasions, leads to a 'resistance to slimming.' We have found no evidence in this group of obese women that weight cycling leads to a progressive decrease in basal metabolic rate or increase in the proportion of body fat." The researchers attributed the reduced amount of weight loss in the second and third cycles to decreased compliance with the diet.

The Cambridge scientists also reviewed fourteen different studies conducted with laboratory rats. None of the studies showed a significant increase in body fat after repetitive episodes of weight gain and weight loss. The researchers described this as "a remarkable consensus that body composition is unaffected by weight cycling."

Their overall conclusion: "The 'dieting makes you fat' theory is regularly reinforced by the lay press and is frequently cited by obese people as a reason for not entering treatment programs. As with many attractive theories, its influence has far exceeded its supporting evidence."

Most studies on yo-yo dieting have been conducted on a retrospective basis. However, scientists at the University of Limburg in Holland in common with the Cambridge group also performed a *prospective* study.

The Dutch trial compared a group of women categorized as yo-yo dieters with another group which did not have a background of repetitive weight loss and weight regain. Over the course of fourteen weeks the patients consumed a diet of 722-840 calories a day and took part in one-hour exercise sessions four times a week. A separate group of non yo-yo dieters did no exercise.

The average weight loss was forty-three pounds and a decrease in resting metabolic rate was noted for all three groups. Interestingly, there was no difference at all between the yo-yo and non yo-yo groups but there was a significantly smaller decline for the exercisers. The benefit of including exercise was also very apparent in burning fat as opposed to lean body mass (a subject which will be discussed in Chapter 20).

Researchers Robert Jeffery, Rena Wing, and Simone French at the University of Minnesota and the University of Pittsburgh compared 101 women and 101 men, all of whom reported a history of back and forth weight loss and weight gain. The researchers tested blood pressure, cholesterol levels, blood sugar, and lean body mass. Their conclusion, published in 1992 in *The American Journal of Clinical Nutrition*: "Our results provide no support for the hypothesis that weight cycling adversely affects body composition, metabolic efficiency, or cardiovascular risk factors. Concerns about the hazards of dieting-related weight fluctuations are at present premature."

Another study, actually entitled "The Myth of the Yo-Yo," was conducted at the University of Cambridge. Scientists there compared four patients, who, eighteen months earlier, had lost substantial amounts of weight on a very low-calorie diet and experienced variable weight regain. The patients were monitored over an eight-week period and the researchers reported "no suggestion of impairment in ability to lose weight."

One major question, overlooked by the critics of yo-yo dieting, is this: What would have happened to the overweight person if he or she had not made repeated attempts to lose weight? There is little research on the subject, but it is more likely than not that these individuals would have become *even heavier*. By not dieting they would almost certainly have stayed on a continuous pattern of weight gain. Ideally, the dieter won't regain but it is better to have lost some weight, even if it is regained, than for the dieter to have continued to do nothing but gain. Ultimately, the yo-yo dieters, in comparison, are at less health risk. So go for it!

## *WHY ARE YOU OVERWEIGHT?*

How did you get so big in the first place? Well, for one thing, you can't choose your parents—and you may well have been genetically handicapped from birth. If both of your parents are overweight, there's a striking 80% chance you will be, too. One overweight parent gives you a 40% likelihood, while with two slim parents your risk is very small, about 10%.

But were you born to be fat? Is it in your genes? Were you overfed as a child and developed a lifetime pattern of overindulgence? Is it eating the wrong kind of food that's to blame, or just eating too much?

There's not one single simple answer to the question of why some of us gain weight more easily than others. Obesity is caused by a complex interaction of genetic, social, cultural, and emotional factors. All the evidence is still not in, but over the last few years fascinating studies in many parts of the world have been coming up with some of the answers.

## *ALL IN THE FAMILY*

Several studies clearly pinpoint a powerful genetic influence. One major survey compared the weight of adopted children with that of their biological and adoptive parents. World renowned obesity researcher Dr. Albert Stunkard, of the University of Pennsylvania, and a team from the University of Texas Health Science

Center, joined forces with a group of Danish investigators to trace 4,500 Danish adoptees born in the 1920s.

They discovered a striking similarity between the size of the biological parents (particularly the mother) and the children (particularly the daughters). There was a direct parallel across the whole range of body shape, from thin to very fat. There was no such relationship between the adoptees and their adoptive parents.

The genetic connection was also demonstrated when Dr. Stunkard, in a study published in the *New England Journal of Medicine* in 1990, disclosed that identical twins ended up as adults with virtually the same body weights whether they were reared apart or together. The weight on nonidentical (fraternal) twins varied much more even when they were raised in the same home.

In another landmark 1990 study, researchers at Laval University in Quebec, Canada, took a different approach by deliberately overfeeding twelve sets of identical twins. The twins—lean young men—were fed a total of an additional 84,000 calories. They overindulged at the rate of an extra 1,000 calories a day, six days a week, over a 100-day period. The twins in each pair gained almost exactly the same amount of weight, and even in the same places. One pair would gain weight in the abdomen; another in the buttocks and thighs. One set of twins gained more than twenty-nine pounds; another set gained only nine-and-a-half pounds. (I'm sure you'll be glad to know that most of the participants who gained weight "in the cause of science" returned to their original weight within six months of returning to their normal diets.)

Says Dr. Stunkard, "What does all of this tell people who are having problems with their weight? It gives them a nonjudgmental, reasonable explanation. It tells them that genetically they've got the dice loaded against them."

David Jonas, of Corpus Christi, Texas, certainly feels that the genetic dice were loaded against him. David, who, over the years, ballooned to 512 pounds, can trace a family history of obesity. His mother, father, and eldest brother all died from the complications of obesity, he says, and the entire family, including seven children, have battled a weight problem.

Recalls David: "I've heard stories of my grandfather, who I never met, and how he weighed well over 300 pounds and went to an early grave. Then there was great aunt Ruth who baked the best six-layer cake in the county. She had no idea how much she weighed and didn't want to know. Her husband tricked her into going with him to the cotton gin in their horse-drawn wagon to weigh his cotton. Later, he went back without her knowledge and weighed the same wagon again, but without her on it. Afterward, everybody but aunt Ruth knew that, at 650 pounds, she weighed more than the bale of cotton. She was buried in a piano crate."

After thirty years of fighting what he thought was a losing battle, David was at his wit's end, and convinced he was going to follow his parents and brother to an early grave. "I felt that perhaps the battle was lost and soon to be over. I was so miserable, mentally and physically, that I wanted to give up and die and stop being such a burden to others. Having tried virtually every approach known to man and having my hopes dashed by all of them, you can understand my skepticism."

David decided to try one more diet and, after losing more than 200 pounds, is a skeptic no more. "To say The Micro Diet has changed my life is like saying the Grand Canyon is just another ditch. The Micro Diet has not just changed my life, it has given my life back to me."

The genetic influence is undoubtedly a powerful one. So, the person who claims he only has to "look at a chocolate to gain a pound," may not be so far from the truth, after all. He may well have been born with a lower metabolic rate and therefore does not burn calories to the same extent as his slim friends.

If you do have a lower metabolic rate it's going to dog you throughout life. Look at the numbers. One pound of fat contains about 3,500 calories. Reducing your food intake by 1,000 calories a day should, therefore, result in weight losses of two pounds a week. However, as soon as you go on a diet, your body reacts defensively and your metabolic rate (the rate at which you burn calories) is further reduced by up to 15%. The result is slower weight loss, making even seven pounds a month difficult to achieve by eliminating as many as 1,000 calories a day from your diet.

This is nature's age-old way of adapting your body to help you in times of famine. It is not, of course, an advantage in modern society, where that "protective" padding of fat no longer has a purpose.

Generally, men lose weight more quickly than women, young people more quickly than old, and large people more quickly than small. This is because of their higher metabolic rate, which makes it easier to produce an energy deficit. A five-foot-tall, 60-year-old woman who is twenty-eight pounds overweight may have a metabolic rate that burns only 1,700 calories a day. To achieve a weight loss of just two pounds a week, her food intake would have to be less than 700 calories a day, low by any standards.

Indeed, Dr. Denis Craddock, a member of the Royal College of Physicians' Working Party on obesity, says, "Some women will, in fact, gain weight on a routine where they are encouraged to eat about 1,500 calories a day."

## *EATING TOO MUCH*

So, yes, to paraphrase Dr. Stunkard, the dice may be loaded against some people from birth. It may be in your genes. You may have been dealt a cruel blow, but that's no reason to sit back and accept your "fate". You may have started life with a definite disadvantage, but at least you know that you have to be particularly careful to avoid gaining extra pounds, and that your children should be on guard, as well.

You may not be overeating compared to other people, but you are overeating in relation to what your own body is burning off. The good news is that studies show that you can overcome your genetic predisposition.

The reality, however, is that many of us just simply overindulge. In effect, the grim message from the Surgeon General's Report was—we're eating ourselves to death. Bluntly declaring that diseases of dietary excess and imbalance were among the leading causes of death in the United States, (accounting for 1.5 million lives a year) the report said, "Overconsumption . . . is now a major concern for Americans."

It added, "What we eat may affect our risk for several of the leading causes of death; notably coronary artery disease, stroke, atherosclerosis, diabetes, and some types of cancer. These disorders together now account for more than two-thirds of all deaths in the United States."

## *EATING THE WRONG KIND OF FOOD*

Despite genetic considerations, *what* we eat, rather than *how much* we eat, may turn out to be the key factor in weight gain. Early findings from the most wide-ranging study ever undertaken of the relationship between diet and the risk of developing health problems certainly point in that direction.

The study, orchestrated by Cornell University scientist Dr. T. Colin Campbell, is monitoring 6,500 people in China. Adjusted for height, the Chinese actually eat and drink 20% more calories than the average American. Yet, Americans are 25% fatter. Why is that? One of the chief causes could be because the Chinese eat only one-third as much fat as Americans, and they eat double the starch.

Eating a lot of protein, particularly animal protein, has also been linked to chronic disease. Americans not only eat a third more protein than Chinese, but 70% of it comes from animal sources compared with but 7% of Chinese protein. Those Chinese people in the study who have adopted an American-style diet, also have the highest rates of heart disease, diabetes, and cancer among Chinese. One of the main conclusions from this massive study is that a plant-based eating plan is more likely to promote good health and less obesity.

But never mind the Chinese, it's Americans who are in trouble. As the 20th century comes to a close, Americans are consuming 31% more fat, 43% less complex carbohydrates, and performing 75% less physical activity than in 1900. And if you want a real shock, consider the eating habits of our paleolithic ancestors. Studies of fossils reveal that cave men ate substantially more dietary fiber a day than do Americans in the 1990s. Our ancestors also ate plenty of lean, wild meat and much less fat, and it goes without saying that they got plenty of exercise.

## *THE SURGEON GENERAL'S REPORT AND THE MICRO DIET*

So how does The Micro Diet compare with the Chinese and caveman diets? How does it stack up against the recommendations in the Surgeon General's report? Well, The Micro Diet fully complies with the major findings of this 712-page report, as well as the recommendations of leading health organizations such as The American Heart Association and The American Cancer Society. Here's how the loser-friendly Micro Diet meets the seven key points of federal nutrition policy as stated in the *Dietary Guidelines for Americans:*

**Eat a Variety of Foods:** The dietary recommendations emphasize consumption of vegetables, fruits, and whole grain products, fish, poultry (prepared without skin), lean meats, and low-fat dairy products. This, of course, is to ensure that the dieter receives all of his or her daily nutritional needs. The Micro Diet accomplishes this by providing nutritionally-fortified meals—such as chili, Spanish rice, pasta, cereals, shakes, soups, and bars—made out of foods such as nonfat milk, egg whites, grains, fruits, and vegetables. They are primarily plant-based foods.

**Maintain Desirable Weight:** That's the principal goal of The Micro Diet program. The meals are ideal not just for the dieter, but anyone interested in maintaining their weight through healthy eating.

**Avoid Too Much Fat, Saturated Fat and Cholesterol:** Dietary fat accounts for about 37% of the total energy intake of Americans, well above the recommended upper limit of 30%. Three or four Micro meals per day provides from as little as 4% of fat calories per day up to a maximum of 29%. It's recommended that saturated fat, which primarily comes from animal products, represent no more than 10% of calories in your diet. Since Micro meals are primarily plant-based foods they contain very little saturated fat. Saturated fat is found in whole milk, but the Micro meals contain nonfat milk. The average American consumes an average of 600 mgs of dietary cholesterol per day while the recommendation is 250 to 300 mgs or less. Many Micro meals have no cholesterol at all and the maximum daily intake for the average dieter using these meals as their sole source of nutrition is likely to be just 11 mgs.

**Eat Foods with Adequate Starch and Fiber:** A daily diet emphasizing foods high in complex carbohydrates and fiber is associated with lower rates of diverticulitis and colon cancer—the second most common form of cancer. It is recommended that carbohydrates form at least 50%–70% of your daily caloric intake and that you consume twenty to thirty grams of fiber a day. All Micro meals contain 50%–70% carbohydrate (including varying measures of complex carbohydrates); some products have a generous amount of fiber (eight grams), while others serve a useful four grams per meal. Some meals, such as the nonfat milk-based drinks have no fiber (you wouldn't expect them to).

For an ongoing diet we recommend that you keep your fat intake low, and fiber intake at the twenty to thirty grams of fiber a day level by combining Micro meals with fruits, vegetables, and whole grains. Fiber consumption in North America today is low: an average of just ten to fifteen grams per day, although most vegetarians consume about thirty-seven grams. What exactly is fiber? Fiber is the skeleton of the plant, without which it would collapse. There are two types, both of which are beneficial to your body: 1) The gummy water-soluble fibers found in oatmeal, beans, bananas, fruits, and vegetables; 2) Water-insoluble fiber, which includes bran, whole grain cereals, and breads.

Can fiber help weight control? There is evidence that it can. Dr. K. W. Heaton, writing in the British medical publication *The Lancet*, showed that eating high-fiber bread as opposed to white bread enabled the body to pass some calories through the system without being absorbed, and to speed that transit by five times or more. His research sparked additional studies at the Department of Food Science and Human Nutrition at Michigan State University. This showed that people on a high-fiber diet voluntarily ate less and appeared to absorb less fat in addition to the weight-loss effect owing to calories being 'passed through' the body. Their report stimulated headlines claiming: The more bread you eat, the more weight you lose.

Fiber can play an important role, too, in reducing the feeling of hunger on a diet program. A study at the University of Copenhagen in Denmark compared two groups. In both groups the men consumed 466 calories a day and the women 388 calories. The only other difference was that one group received thirty grams a day of plant fiber. The two groups had similar weight losses—twenty-two pounds over four weeks—but when fiber was added, hunger ratings were significantly lower.

The evidence for inclusion of adequate dietary fiber is persuasive, therefore, as part of a long-term weight maintenance program, but like everything else in life there needs to be a balance. Too much fiber causes the body to fail to absorb some essential minerals, especially zinc. So how to obtain sufficient fiber? Listed here are some of the most common sources.

## *FOODS TO PROVIDE 23g DIETARY FIBER PER DAY*

**Fruit group:** About 2g fiber per serving; use four or more per day. About 60 calories per serving.

| | |
|---|---|
| Apple, 1 small | Orange, 1 small |
| Banana, 1 small | Peach, 1 medium |
| Strawberries, ½ cup | Pear, ½ small |
| Cherries, 10 large | Plums, 2 small |

**Bread and cereal group:** About 2g fiber per serving; use four or more per day. About 80 calories per serving.

| | |
|---|---|
| Whole-wheat bread, 1 slice | All Bran, 1 tablespoon |
| Rye bread, 1 slice | Corn Flakes, ⅔ cup |
| Cracked wheat bread, 1 slice | Oatmeal, dry, 3 tablespoons |
| Shredded wheat, ½ biscuit | Wheat Bran, 1 teaspoon |
| Grape-Nuts, 3 tablespoons | Puffed Wheat, 1½ cups |

**Vegetable group:** About 2g fiber per serving; use four or more per day. About 25 calories per serving. These values are for cooked portions.

| | |
|---|---|
| Broccoli, ½ stalk | Lettuce, raw, 2 cups |
| Brussels sprouts, 4 | Green beans, ½ cup |
| Carrots, ⅓ cup | Potato, 2-inch diameter |
| Celery, 1 cup | Tomato, raw, 1 medium |
| Corn on the cob, 2-inch piece | Baked beans, canned, 2 tablespoons |

**Miscellaneous group:** About 1g fiber per serving.

| | |
|---|---|
| Peanut butter, 2½ teaspoons | Pickle, 1 large |

SOURCE: Adapted from "Recommendation for a High-fiber Diet," *Nutrition and the MD,* July 1981.

**Micro meals group:**

| | | |
|---|---|---|
| Peanut Bar | 8 grams | 260 calories |
| Muesli Cereal | 8 grams | 260 calories |
| Muesli Bar | 6 grams | 280 calories |
| Chocolate Bar | 5 grams | 280 calories |
| Chili | 4 grams | 210 calories |
| Yogurt-Orange Bar | 4 grams | 290 calories |
| Crunchy Peanut Bar | 4 grams | 290 calories |
| Popcorn Bar | 3 grams | 290 calories |
| Spanish Rice | 2 grams | 260 calories |
| Tomato Soup | 1 gram | 244 calories |

In practice, of course, you would be eating a mixture of foods to provide enough fiber, and you can probably rely on your current diet to provide at least half of what you need, especially if you are eating from the above list. By studying the above you can devise your own low-calorie/high-fiber plan. Alternatively, you can add natural bran to breakfast cereal, yogurt, or hamburgers or, of course, one of your glasses of Micro drinks.

**Avoid Too Much Sugar:** Too much sugar in the diet contributes to obesity, and eaten between meals contributes toward cavities. But some sugar in the diet can go a long way toward enhancing the flavor of a low-fat diet. Taste is of critical importance to the dieter. Some Micro meals such as the drinks and soups contain no sugar at all but, as The Micro Diet is definitely not designed to be a Spartan regimen, some of our meals, e.g. the bars, do contain sugar. However, the calorie level of Micro meals is so low the amount of sugar is not excessive compared to an individual's normal daily intake.

**Avoid Too Much Sodium:** Sodium is highly necessary for normal metabolic function but the sodium intake of adults in the United States is in the range of four to six grams per day, far beyond the 1.1 to 3.3 grams per day recommended by the National Research Council as "safe and adequate." Micro meals contain from as little as 85 mgs per serving up to a maximum of 850 mgs. The average daily consumption for most people would be 1.2 grams per day making The Micro Diet a LOW-sodium regime.

**If You Drink Alcoholic Beverages, Do So in Moderation:**
Agreed. It would be particularly unwise for anyone on the 800-calorie-a-day program to consume alcohol, as it would just "go to your head."

## *ARE YOU READY?*

Chances are that you've dieted before—and failed to keep the weight off. You probably have a good idea why you became overweight in the first place, and why you're still overweight. The loser-friendly Micro Diet makes it possible for you to achieve the goal of getting down to your ideal weight and, of greater importance, to achieve lasting success.

As you strive to gain control over your life and health, you can benefit from the examples of successful dieters who once felt as hopeless as you may today. People such as Muff Juber, of Renton, Washington, who lost over 100 pounds in just six months; Sal Serio, of Port St. Lucie, Florida, whose ninety-two pound weight loss led to a fabulous new career helping other people lose weight and lead healthier lifestyles; executive chef Bill McLeish, who gained ninety-four pounds thanks to his own cooking, and got rid of it the loser-friendly way; Suzanne de Rham, of Ormond Beach, Florida, who shed twenty-two pounds, and slips again into the swimsuit she wore thirty-three years ago when she was first runner-up in the Miss Kentucky contest; and many, many more.

You know the health hazards of being overweight. You know the benefits of losing your excess weight, even if you have been a yo-yo dieter. The full-spectrum Micro Diet program is the modern answer to long-term weight management, but it's really up to you. Whatever amount you need to lose, you have to acknowledge that fact. You then have your target. And then you must make a commitment! You must want to win the battle over your weight problem as much as the Olympic athlete wants the gold medal. Don't just read this book. Be prepared to take action and win your "gold."

## ■ A CASE STUDY

### BEVERLY FUNK AND PATTI CARLSON: A FAMILY WINS BY LOSING

The mother and daughter dieting team of Beverly Funk and Patti Carlson have together lost 180 pounds, and kept it off.

Patti lost 105 pounds and dropped from a size twenty-four pants to size eight over four years ago. Subsequently, while having her second child, she regained some weight and is now back to her ideal size and shape. Says thirty-year-old Patti, of Bloomingdale, Illinois, "I tend to be an emotional eater. If I get upset about anything, I immediately reach for food. I also eat out of boredom. I love being a housewife and full-time mother, but when my eight-year-old goes to school and my little one goes for a nap, it's difficult for me not to walk into the kitchen and start eating just for something to do."

Patti went on The Micro Diet following the recommendation of her doctor and was ahead of her mother in the losing stakes. "What I did to encourage my mother, so that she didn't have to keep going out and buying new clothes as she lost the weight, was to give her the next size down that she needed from my own wardrobe. Now she's even walking around in jeans and slacks," says Patti.

Patti maintains her weight of 138 pounds by using Micro meals once or twice a day as part of her lifestyle. If she finds that a few extra pounds have crept back on, she uses The Micro Diet again as her sole source of nutrition. "This is the first time since I was in seventh grade that I have been able to keep my weight off for any length of time. I am amazed at how easy it has been. It just blows my mind when I think about the fact that I've gone from a size twenty-four pants to a size eight. Every time I do the laundry and I'm pulling my clothes out of the dryer, I think, 'This thing fits me?' I always dreamed about wearing small sizes and all my tops are now small. I never in my lifetime thought I'd ever see that.

"My life has improved one hundred percent. The Micro Diet has dramatically changed my life and it seems to get better every day. I wouldn't be the person I am today without The Micro Diet. I know I wouldn't have been able to keep my weight off with any other diet because I tried all other kinds. It's very scary to think that I could still weigh what I used to and be sitting on the couch eating bon bons, watching my life go by without enjoying it. I have a different mind-set about so many things. For instance, if we're invited to a party or wedding, I can't wait to go out and buy new clothes. When I was overweight I didn't even want to go to the event, let alone think about what I could wear."

Losing weight together, she says, has created an even closer bond with her mother. "We love to go shopping together. Once upon a time, getting mom to the mall was like taking her to a dentist. Now I can't get her out of the clothes stores. She's worse than I am. We both wear the same size now, so we can trade. We bowl together. We power walk together. We've just become closer and closer because we can do all the things that thin people do. We don't have to wear tents anymore and we can wear belts on our waists."

Mom agrees. Beverly, who lives half an hour from Patti in Franklin Park, Illinois, says; "I'm proud to have a figure again and to be able to buy sixes and eights off the rack in any store. I have a whole new lifestyle. I once was a couch potato but now I go bowling, roller skating, gardening, and do all sorts of activities with family and friends. I exercise daily. I know that I am in charge and have the freedom to choose what to eat, where to eat, when to eat, and with whom to eat."

Beverly, who lost seventy-five pounds in six months, now weighs 130 pounds, a weight she has maintained for three-and-a-half years. Like Patti, she continues to use Micro meals as part of her everyday eating plan. "I have learned to live and forgive myself for mistakes and therefore I give myself a boundary of three to five pounds to gain. When that happens I go back on The Micro Diet as my exclusive source of food to take it off in a few days."

Beverly describes herself as a yo-yo dieter who lost weight on numerous diets and then regained it. "I was like a roly-poly caterpillar who went into a cocoon every winter and emerged even fatter. I lived a life of making excuses: I was never too fat, just not tall enough or pleasingly plump. I hated shopping because I didn't want to look at myself in the mirror, so I ordered out of catalogues."

Today, when presented with the temptation of food, Beverly asks herself, "Do I want this sweet roll, pizza, or piece of cake, or do I want to look, feel, and be who I am now?" Usually the answer is the latter, but sometimes Beverly elects to "indulge." "The Micro Diet is a forgiving diet. I have learned to appreciate the fact that it's O.K. to make 'mistakes' and then go right back on The Micro Diet, rather than feel like a failure, punishing myself, and continuing to gain all the weight back. I now have control over food, I don't let food control me. I've maintained my weight and I know in my heart this is the weight I'll be forever. The Micro Diet gives everyone a chance to be slim for life, and it works for all ages."

# 3

# THE BREAKTHROUGH

THE SEARCH FOR THE perfect diet has challenged researchers for decades. The lack of a clear-cut solution to the problem of obesity has, of course, led to fierce debate within the scientific community, and also enabled unqualified opportunists to promote a wide range of weight-loss schemes from the really ridiculous to the downright dangerous.

Over the years crash "starvation" has gone through a period of being in vogue, while today many dietitians still recommend the "traditional" moderate approach of about 1,200 calories intake a day. Both programs have their drawbacks. Fasting can cause serious health problems—even death. And, for many people, the weight loss on a 1,200-calorie plan is so slow that they become dispirited and give up.

One of the key reasons that this 1,200-calorie barrier has existed is simply because dietitians were concerned that dieters would not obtain sufficient nutrition on fewer calories. But one of the problems is that the dieter often miscalculates the portion sizes and consumes even more than 1,200 calories. This "magic" number was also established, of course, before the discovery of many nutrients, and before the advent of specially formulated meals fortified with all of the required vitamins and minerals. The 1,200-calorie barrier made sense twenty years ago; it doesn't make sense today.

Conversely, when "meal replacements" were popularized in the early 1980s, they were usually very low-calorie plans of 300 to 400 calories per day. They had the advantage of providing complete nutrition and took the question of portion control out of the hands of the dieter. Indeed, when The Micro Diet was originally introduced a decade ago it fell into this category but, in view of the latest research, has evolved to become a program which promotes a minimum of 800 calories a day as part of a full-spectrum approach to weight management, including lifestyle modification, exercise, and personal support. A *very* low-calorie plan made sense ten years ago; it doesn't make sense today. That's why The Micro Diet is now a low-calorie plan.

I will fully explain the rationale later in this chapter, but first let's review the sixty years of scientific research which has brought us to this conclusion, beginning with the original very low-calorie experiments. These were performed as long ago as the 1930s when a group of American doctors devised 400–600 calorie a day diets using conventional food. Although the diet was deficient in some nutrients, it was reasonably well-balanced and the results were successful. Over 300 patients monitored by researchers Strang, McClugage, and Evans at the Western Pennsylvania Hospital in Pittsburgh, lost an average of twenty-two pounds over eight weeks with no ill effects.

In spite of their triumphs, they did not pursue their studies further, and it was to be years before anyone else took up the research. The next stage, actually, was a backward one, when fasting went through a phase of popularity in the late 1950s and early 1960s. It is difficult today to comprehend why such 'zero calorie–zero nutrition' programs were promoted. Not surprisingly, spectacular weight losses were achieved but the body's vital organs were placed at serious risk and, in fact, such diets led to deaths, even with hospital patients under constant medical supervision.

In the mid-60s, very low-calorie, high-protein regimens were explored, primarily by Dr. Robert E. Bolinger at the University of Kansas and, in France, by Dr. Marian Apfelbaum of the University of Paris. Another of the early pioneers, Dr. George Blackburn at the Center for Nutritional Research in Boston, developed a program in which four ounces of lean meat, fish, or fowl were consumed three times a day, and he coined the term "Protein Sparing Modified Fast."

In the early 1970s researchers on both sides of the Atlantic, Doctors Saul Genuth and Victor Vertes at Mount Sinai Medical Center in Cleveland, and Doctors Alan Howard and Ian McLean

Baird in Cambridge and London, respectively, were independently discovering the advantages of adding carbohydrates to the very low-calorie regimen.

Reporting on their experience with more than 500 patients, the Cleveland scientists concluded, "Supplemented fasting can be accomplished with safety and efficiency on a large-scale outpatient basis," and "is now recognized as an effective means of achieving substantial weight loss rapidly and safely with a minimum of patient discomfort."

Tragically, and scandalously, the commercial marketing of a very low-calorie "liquid protein" diet, which had not been subjected to clinical trials, cast a dark cloud over all of this groundbreaking work. Popularized in the United States in 1977 and 1978 as "The Last Chance Diet," these products contained collagen, a low-quality protein lacking certain essential amino acids; they contained no carbohydrate; and were also deficient in potassium—a highly necessary element for the heart to function properly. A large number of deaths were attributed to the "liquid protein" plan owing to heart problems, and the diet, quite rightly, was banned.

This whole sorry episode had a serious impact on the acceptance of very low-calorie diets. Some tenacious researchers, however, would not give up. Convinced of the validity of this approach, they continued to study the benefits of formulations that included **all** of the essential nutrients and **a balance** of protein, carbohydrate, and fat. In the United States, the work of Genuth and Vertes led to the development of the Optifast program, while in Great Britain, the research of Howard and McLean Baird created The Cambridge Diet. Both programs provided little more than 300 calories a day: the American version was high-protein; the British investigators preferred a high-carbohydrate approach.

Time and again, all of these independent researchers found their patients losing weight rapidly—just as quickly as they would on a dangerous starvation plan but without the serious side effects. On the contrary, significant health improvements were noted:

- Cholesterol and triglyceride levels dropped for those patients with high levels.
- Hypertensive patients noticed a dramatic drop in blood pressure.
- Diabetics, too, recorded beneficial lowering of blood glucose.

The most comprehensive and independent assessment of the effectiveness and safety of very low-calorie diets was reported in one of the world's foremost medical journals, *The Annals of Internal Medicine*, which is published by the American College of Physicians. Written by a team from the University of Pennsylvania, Doctors Thomas Wadden, Albert Stunkard, and Kelly Brownell, all major researchers in the field of obesity, it reported safe, average weight losses of fifteen to twenty-two pounds in a month and at least forty-four pounds over twelve weeks.

Their conclusions: "As contrasted to the earlier 'liquid protein' diets that were associated with at least sixty deaths, very low-calorie diets of high-quality protein appear safe when limited to three months or less under careful medical supervision." The safety evidence, they stated, came from round-the-clock monitoring of heart action and the fact that no diet-related fatalities had been reported in over 10,000 cases.

### Effectiveness

Weight losses are "far greater" than for other nonsurgical treatments, such as behavior modification, diet, and anorectic drugs, said the Pittsburgh-based researchers. They reported that only 10% of patients treated with conventional therapies *ever* achieve a weight loss of forty-four pounds. That's the *average* weight loss for just twelve weeks on a very low-calorie diet.

### Safety

Diuretics are often used to treat patients with high blood pressure, sometimes with serious side effects. The Pennsylvania doctors suggested very low-calorie diets "may be safer than diuretic agents in the treatment of hypertension in the obese."

The survey authors then turned their attention to heart function since, with the grossly inadequate liquid protein diets, heart irregularities were found to be the principal health hazard. Their assessment: "Cardiac performance is not adversely affected by very low-calorie diets of high-quality protein; in fact it may actually be improved."

### The future

The researchers concluded: "Large rapid weight losses and reductions in risk factors make the use of very low-calorie diets attractive.... Attention must be directed to the problem of maintenance of weight losses. A comprehensive program combining very low-calorie diets (to achieve a large initial weight loss) with nutrition education, exercise, training, and behavior modification would appear to be the next step."

The loser-friendly Micro Diet is that next step. Since the publication of the Pennsylvania review, many more clinical trials have been conducted involving tens of thousand of patients under rigorous medical supervision. Over the years I have monitored all of this scientific research, discussed the results with doctors and other health professionals and, of course, listened to the feedback from dieters in many countries.

Today's loser-friendly Micro Diet has evolved out of a careful analysis of all of the clinical studies and real-life experiences. There is now overwhelming evidence to support:

- 800 calories a day, rather than a very low-calorie diet.
- Solid, prepared meals, rather than a liquid-only approach.
- A balance of protein and carbohydrate, rather than a high–low mix.

## *THE ROAD TO 800 CALORIES*

The original Micro Diet program, tested in the early 1980s at the University of Surrey in England and at the University of Utrecht in Holland, reflected the thinking at that time that a very low-calorie program was "the answer." This was a 330-calorie-a-day plan providing forty-two grams of protein.

The University of Surrey study produced average weight losses of sixteen pounds a month and led senior lecturer in nutrition, Dr. B. Jacqueline Stordy, to observe, "Patients enjoy a sense of well-being...their weight loss is so rewarding. It doesn't take a lifetime to lose a substantial amount. The Micro Diet actually gives dieters a sense of freedom because they can go out and enjoy themselves socially or for business, and then go back on the diet and quickly start losing again. This diet is the answer for anyone who has had real difficulty losing weight."

Dr. Stordy's comments are echoed by the medical doctor who supervised the trial, Dr. John Wright, reader in metabolic medicine at the university, "I have no hesitation in saying that for people with a low metabolic rate this is an extremely effective and, above all, realistic new approach."

The trial at the University of Utrecht was deliberately conducted with women who were only slightly overweight, yet still showed an average weight loss of eleven pounds in fourteen days. Says Dr. Anton Beynen, the physician in charge, "A well-formulated regimen such as The Micro Diet is undoubtedly the diet of the future. It solves all the previous problems because patients lose weight fast enough to be encouraged and they feel very well at the same time."

Subsequent tests at the University of Barcelona in Spain with a 500-calorie, sixty grams of protein plan; and at the University of Heidelberg in Germany with a 660-calorie, fifty grams of protein program, provided us with a fascinating result. The 660-calorie diet produced:

1. The fastest and biggest weight loss—19.2 pounds in a month—in fact, an unbroken steady weight loss over the whole thirty-day trial.
2. No hunger among the dieters involved.
3. A significant reduction in blood pressure.
4. An average decrease in cholesterol levels of 26%.
5. An average 38% drop in triglyceride levels, i.e., the levels of fat circulating in blood.

Why did the 660-calorie diet produce a higher weight loss than the 330-calorie program? The dieters were heavier to begin with, which certainly helped. But it's highly likely that the 660-calorie dieters were adhering to the diet, while the 330-calorie dieters, says cardiologist Dr. Alfred Wirth who conducted the trial, weren't satisfied on such a low-calorie intake and were, in reality, adding a lot more calories.

The frequently recommended 1,200-calorie level is too high to produce a weight loss that is motivating enough to keep many dieters faithful to the diet, says Dr. Wirth, adding that a calorie level needs to be "high enough to allow the dieter to get enough protein and to feel satisfied" and yet "low enough to produce an encouragingly fast weight loss."

More recently, other research has clearly shown that 800 calories a day also achieves the same kind of significant weight losses as lower intakes. A study published in 1992 in *The American Journal of Clinical Nutrition* reported on a trial conducted at the Universities of Pennsylvania and Syracuse which compared the benefits of 420-, 600-, and 880-calorie-a-day diets.

Seventy-six overweight women were randomly assigned, without their knowledge, to one of the three regimens for twelve weeks. This was followed by a further six weeks during which time conventional foods were gradually reintroduced, until all of the dieters were consuming 1,000 calories a day. Average weight loss after the twelve-week low-calorie dieting period was thirty-nine pounds and, after the eighteen-week period, forty-five pounds. In all three programs fat comprised at least 85% of the weight lost with dieters reporting significant and comparable decreases in hunger.

The authors commented, "The study's most important finding is that there were no significant differences in weight losses or changes in body composition."

The researchers speculated that this was attributable to a combination of reasons: dieters on the lower caloric intake not "sticking to" the plan, as well as variances in the metabolic rate of the dieters. Their conclusion: in effect, no need to reduce caloric intake below 800 calories. The results from an 800-calorie-a-day diet are just as good as from a 420-calorie plan!

The same conclusion was reached by Harvard Medical School researchers, led by Dr. George Blackburn, after a study which involved 1,429 dieters, who had either embarked on a 420-calorie-a-day diet or an 800-calorie-a-day diet along with behavior therapy sessions and mild exercise. Despite the 380-calorie-a-day difference, the rate of weight loss between the two groups was no different.

They reported "clinically and statistically significant health benefits were observed for patients with hypertension and diabetes."

Says Dr. Blackburn, "There's no reason for the diet to be less than 650 to 800 calories a day because the body will just slow its metabolism to adjust."

A British study with 108 overweight women produced similar results. Researchers J. S. Garrow and J. D. Webster from the Clinical Research Centre, Harrow, and the Medical College of St. Bartholomew's Hospital, London, closely monitored the dieters in a metabolic ward. In twenty-one days, consuming 800 calories a day, the patients lost an average of eleven pounds. One woman actually shed a staggering twenty-eight pounds, but it is speculated that water constituted a significant part of her weight loss.

**The Loser-Friendly program, therefore, recommends a minimum daily intake of 800 calories.**

## *PROTEIN VS. CARBOHYDRATE*

The amount and quality of protein in one's diet has long been a subject of controversy, especially since the popularity of the "liquid protein" diets in the 1970s and The Cambridge Diet, in the early 1980s, which originally contained just thirty-five grams of protein a day. As discussed earlier, studies show that high-quality protein provides safe weight loss, and to ensure appropriate fat loss rather than lean body tissue, most researchers insist that the dieter consumes the RDA for protein, fifty-six grams for men and forty-four grams for women.

Major researcher Professor Hans Ditschuneit, of Ulm University, Germany, proved that when weight was lost on a very low-calorie diet the loss was 79% fat, 18% water, and 3% protein. This is significant because when weight is gained, an average 75% of the gain is fat, 19% is water, and 6% extra protein. Some protein loss is inevitable since, with weight loss, there is a decrease in skin, connective tissue, supporting structure, and some muscle.

Muscle mass was also shown to be protected on a 500-calorie-a-day diet containing sixty grams of protein. In this University of Antwerp study, dieters lost 31.7 pounds in over six weeks. Highly significant decreases were observed for body weight, body mass index (minus 5.2), and fat weight, whereas lean body mass remained unchanged.

**The Loser-Friendly program recommends that men select meals which serve at least fifty-six grams of protein per day. Women should ensure that they receive forty-four grams.**

## *LIQUIDS VS. SOLIDS*

Liquid-only preparations have been promoted on the grounds that—without the temptation of solid food—dieters were better able to adhere to the diet. However, researchers at the University of Pennsylvania found that dieters on a liquid 420-calorie-a-day diet were hungrier than dieters eating solid food at the same calorie level. The same researchers subsequently compared dieters on a 500-calorie-a-day program (including lean meat, fish, and fowl) with dieters eating a balanced diet of 1,200 calories (including lean meat, fish, fowl, fruits, vegetables, breads, and cereals). Those "deprived" dieters on the low-calorie regime were less hungry, less preoccupied with eating, and, best of all, lost significantly more weight.

**The Loser-Friendly program incorporates a wide range of prepared meals suitable for all dining occasions, including dinner entrees and meal bars.**

So why the loser-friendly Micro Diet program? After all, there are other nutritionally complete low-calorie diets and meal replacements. There are also the heavily advertised commercial diet centers and their packaged meals. Here's why:

Very low-calorie diets did gain a bad reputation in the 60s and 70s. Today these programs are widely accepted as safe and effective, provided they are made available with careful medical supervision and as part of a multidisciplinary approach involving exercise and behavior modification sessions with attendance required at a hospital or clinic. Most of these programs are usually liquid-only, and expensive. And when the diet is over, you return to "regular" food. The commercial diet centers make you pay an upfront fee and insist on weekly visits (during "office hours") to purchase their expensive foods. What's the alternative? You could turn instead to over-the-counter meal replacements which have become popular because of their ready availability and celebrity-heavy promotional campaigns, but most of them are not nutritionally complete (unless milk is added); they cannot replace all of your daily meals and, of course, do not come with a support system.

On the other hand, The Micro Diet provides a variety of nutritionally complete "real meals" for all eating occasions, and does not require medical supervision (unless you have a health problem). You don't have to check in at a storefront facility or clinic, as the meals can be delivered to your own home, and you can choose the kind of personalized support and encouragement that suits you (see Chapter Nine, The Helping Hand). You also have the benefit of a multidimensional, fun, motivating lifestyle modification and exercise program.

It is important to note that The Micro Diet is based on the same scientific research which substantiates the expensive hospital-based programs, yet makes that concept available and affordable for everyone through lay advisors who have already experienced the benefits of the program themselves.

## ■ A CASE STUDY

### MARY BRADFORD: THE PROMISE OF A FULL LIFE

Mary Bradford weighed over 500 pounds. She had been overweight all of her life, she says, and was virtually bedridden—until a 115-pound weight loss with The Micro Diet turned her life around.

Mary, of Boise, Idaho, blames her massive weight gain on the Irish love of chinaware! As she explains, "For generations Irish ladies have aspired to begin marriage with a fine set of porcelain, always decorated with bunches of flowers, enormous roses, bouquets of red and pink blossoms, on the rims, in the center. Then, the proud cook's goal was to cover every petal on the plate with food; mounds of mashed potatoes, massive chunks of meats, and carrots or peas. If a leaf or flower showed on the surface, it would immediately be covered with rich, creamy gravy or sauce. Then the diner would be urged to eat every bit until the beauty of the plate showed through."

The plate had to be wiped clean with the aid of freshly baked bread, and the entire meal washed down with generous cups of milky, sugar-laden tea, always with the admonition to "remember the famine." Food was an expression of "love, security, and home," but it lead to weight gain and the attendant problems of ridicule and ill health. Says Mary, "I will never forget the neighborhood children chanting, 'fatty, fatty, two-by-four,' or my stepmother telling me, 'You are going to be as enormous as all of the women on your dad's side of the family.'"

The eating habits ingrained in the 1930s and '40s have followed her for the rest of her life, and as a result she says she recently "celebrated" her golden anniversary: fifty years of being fat, "fifty years of sporadic dieting and giving up hope." Riddled with osteoarthritis, weighing over 500 pounds and no longer able to walk, she tried group-oriented programs of every kind. Says Mary, "One of the horrors was trying to join Weight Watchers and having a 'private weigh-in' become a public spectacle as the weighers made a big fuss because the scales could not handle my weight. Well, I slunk out of that meeting as quickly as someone my girth could slink, only to be discouraged enough to gain more weight."

Suddenly, after all these fat-shrouded years she found The Micro Diet. "I couldn't walk and The Micro Diet was literally brought to me. I was ashamed and unhappy with my appearance, but I had a loving and understanding Advisor who was full of encouragement. I never stuck to liquid diets or rabbit food for any amount of time but it was obvious to me that with the full line of delicious meals, this was a program I could do. I made up my mind that fifty years was enough and that I owed my husband a wife half my size and twice the companion. I didn't want to be glamorously thin, just healthy, and ordinarily svelte."

Mary embarked on the program and lost seventy-six pounds in less than three months. "I've never suffered a moment's deprivation. I breakfast on cups of coffee and usually an orange-yogurt Micro bar, which tastes like frosted orange cake. Sometimes, I'll have a crunchy peanut bar instead. Since I have difficulty carrying things, with a cane occupying one hand, the Micro bars are the most convenient for me, right now. That means my lunch tends to be a diet soft drink and a chocolate bar. Imagine a slimming lunch of a cake and brownie! It's almost beyond my comprehension that meals like these can aid my weight loss and still be completely nutritious, but they are."

At dinnertime, Mary says her quandary is whether to choose a chili or pasta dish, and she has them served in an attractive crystal bowl. "I'm going to keep the Micro meals as part of my life, with no regrets. A choice of any three meals gives me complete nutrition without my having to do excessive computations or buy special ingredients. I know I am following a sensible, healthy regimen.

"For the first time in fifty years, I can say I not only feel healthier and more energetic, I face the future with confidence that I can be an attractive and well person. I've already gone from being bedridden, to using a walker, then to using a cane, and now even walking a few steps. I want to be small enough to have the knee replacement surgery I need. I want to join my husband on trips and bird-watching expeditions. I want to do my own grocery shopping, pick up things that have fallen on the floor, and choose pretty clothes. Most of all I want to be able to live long enough to enjoy retirement with the husband who has stuck with me through thick and now (hopefully) thin. I know I am on the path to a full and lasting success."

# 4

# THE MEDICAL BENEFITS

THERE IS ABSOLUTELY NO DOUBT that a wide range of health problems can be improved—and resolved—as a result of getting rid of excess fat. The clinical evidence is overwhelming and is supported by every leading health organization in the country.

The authoritative Surgeon General's Report, noting that one-fourth of American adults are overweight and nearly one-tenth are severly overweight, commented, "The extraordinarily high prevalence of obesity in the United States, coupled with its role as a risk factor for diabetes, hypertension, coronary heart disease and stroke, gallbladder disease and some forms of cancer, suggests that a reduction in the average weight of the general population would improve the nation's health. Americans, in general, would benefit from a lifestyle that includes more physical activity and a diet containing fewer calories."

Data from the Framingham Heart Study, published in 1992, reporting on a twenty-six year follow-up of 5,209 men and women showed that the amount of weight gained was a clear indicator of heart disease risk—especially in women. Numerous smaller studies have produced the same findings: The heavier you are, the more likely you are to have a heart attack.

*The Loser-Friendly Diet* gives you the kind of lifestyle recommended by the Surgeon General, and shows you how to make it easy to follow that lifestyle by incorporating low-calorie meals, the concept which has already aided millions of overweight patients around the globe.

Researchers in virtually every European and Scandinavian

country and in other parts of the world as far-flung as Israel, Japan, and Czechoslovakia, have now conducted clinical trials with a variety of very low-calorie diets and low-calorie diets. From these studies, one dominant theme emerges: There is no better way to lose weight and improve your health. Day in and day out, the clinical research is being substantiated by physicians in the field who, in many instances, specifically used The Micro Diet themselves before recommending the program to their patients. Here are the key points from just a few of the more important medical studies conducted on a broad range of very low-calorie diets and low-calorie diets with observations from the clinical researchers involved. The results are applicable to the loser-friendly Micro Diet. You'll also find enthusiastic comments of doctors from across the U.S. who are now implementing The Micro Diet program on an everyday basis.

## *SAFE AND EFFECTIVE*

In one of the largest studies conducted, researcher Marvin A. Kirschner and his colleagues at hospital and university clinics in New Jersey monitored the use of a liquid-only, nutritionally complete, 420-calorie-a-day diet combined with low-intensity aerobic exercise, weekly support, and educational sessions.

Over 4,000 patients took part in this eight-year study, which was published in the *International Journal of Obesity.* Men lost an average of five pounds per week, totalling sixty-six pounds over a thirteen-week period; women lost on average at least three pounds per week resulting in a mean weight loss of forty-seven pounds over a fourteen-week period.

### *High Blood Pressure*

Eighty-three percent of those patients with high blood pressure saw their blood pressure return to normal, and 71% were able to discontinue medication.

### *Diabetes Mellitus*

Of those patients with Type II maturity onset Diabetes Mellitus, 100% were able to discontinue oral hypoglycemics. Of those Type II diabetics requiring insulin injections, 87% were weaned off insulin entirely; the remainder were able to greatly decrease the daily dosage.

### *Hyperlipidemia*

Seventy-seven percent of subjects with high triglyceride and high cholesterol levels found the levels reduced to normal, and lowered in the remainder.

### *Cardiac function*

The heart condition of patients was carefully monitored. Among the 4,000 dieters, there were only three documented instances of non-fatal cardiac arrhythmias.

### *In summary*

The researchers concluded that "using high quality protein supplement and multidisciplinary counselling provides a reasonable success rate for achieving and maintaining weight loss in the morbidly obese population."

## *DOCTORS SPEAK OUT*

Dr. Thomas Green, a gynecologist in Lees Summit, Missouri, appreciates the health-enhancing qualities of such a program, not only for his patients but also for himself, having personally dropped fifty pounds with a very low-calorie diet. He says, "In a short period of time I've lost an incredible amount of weight. It has been a literal lifesaver for me. I've thrown away blood pressure medications and lowered my cholesterol. I now run or walk four or five miles a day, and I'm thankful I'm still around to enjoy my practice, my patients, and my family."

Dr. Green says that he now prefers to use the low-calorie Micro Diet for weight maintenance, and for weight loss recommends it to his patients without hesitation. "It provides rapid and safe weight loss, so people lose quickly and have the motivation to continue. It tastes very good and there's plenty of variety, but what's important to many of my patients is that it is economical."

The motivational helping hand of the lay advisor, he feels, is an essential element contributing to the success of the diet. "The support system is key and is especially useful to involve other dieters. They can really help each other, talking about their progress and exercising together." The Micro Diet, says Dr. Green, is now part of his lifestyle, "I'm using it as more of a maintenance program, but if I go on a trip or holiday and gain a few pounds I use The Micro Diet full time to get the weight back down to where I like it."

Another gynecologist, Dr. Raymond O. Keltner, of Kansas City, Missouri, who has been a practicing M.D. for forty-one years, says that he is delighted to have finally found a weight management program he can wholeheartedly recommend to his patients. "It's far better than anything else I have ever seen before. It's safe and it is effective," he says. "I see many patients struggling with their weight, including those who have just had a baby, and I am very confident putting them on The Micro Diet because of its nutritional composition. Many patients are skeptical at the beginning and say that the diet sounds too good to be true, until they start experiencing weight losses of fourteen pounds a month, feeling good, and having plenty of energy.

"From my standpoint, there isn't much advantage in losing weight if the patient doesn't keep it off, and this is the best program that I have seen for weight maintenance. The program has invaluable elements such as lifestyle modification, exercise, and the motivating Advisor support system. To keep the weight off, I recommend that the patient continues eating Micro meals as part of their everyday lifestyle. That's what I do myself. I personally lost eight pounds in two weeks and I've been using the meals ever since, once or twice a day, because it's convenient, they taste so good, and I know I'm getting great nutrition."

Adds Dr. Keltner, "I see this as an opportunity for many physicians to help get their patients' weight under control and thereby take a major role in reducing health problems such as hypertension, heart disease, diabetes, and other ailments."

## *EFFECTS ON THE HEART*

Researchers at the University of Rochester, led by Dr. Dean Lockwood, have studied the effects of low-calorie diets on the heart. In a series of important studies they proved that, contrasted with the ill-fated "liquid protein" diets of the 1970s, low-calorie, nutritionally complete programs do not cause cardiac arrhythmias.

These doctors monitored patients in a metabolic ward for as long as forty-eight days, including twenty-four-hour electrocardiographic recordings. Their conclusion: "A hypocaloric diet vigorously supplemented with essential elements, micro-nutrients and vitamins appears to be safer than the once popular incomplete liquid protein preparations."

The longest study to date monitoring the effects of a very low-calorie diet on the heart compared the results with dieters on a 1,200-calorie-a-day program.

In the study conducted at the University of Pennsylvania School of Medicine, one group of women ate a 1,200-calorie-a-day diet for forty-five weeks; another group consumed 420 calories a day for the first sixteen weeks before switching to 1,200 calories for the remaining twenty-nine weeks. A group of nondieters was also monitored. At the end of the forty-five-week period, the nondieters had gained an average of 8.6 pounds, the 1,200-calorie dieters had lost an average of 31.9 pounds, and the dieters who initially used the low-calorie approach got rid of 49.3 pounds each.

The researchers found that there are likely to be occasional minor cardiac abnormalities in both dieters and nondieters. In fact, there was a greater incidence of premature heartbeats in the people on the 1,200-calorie diet and the nondieters as opposed to the people on the 420-calorie plan, although the differences were not statistically significant.

That kind of research impressed fellow cardiologist Dr. Donald Fowell, who thoroughly investigated The Micro Diet after his wife, Violet, decided she wanted to follow the program. Now, after seeing the positive results with many patients who had repeatedly failed on other diets, he's more than impressed—he's enthusiastic, too.

Says Dr. Fowell, of Stockton, California, "The Micro Diet is a tool by which we can almost guarantee that people will lose weight, will be able to stay with the program, and can achieve their goal with safety."

Dr. Fowell's convictions about The Micro Diet heightened after seeing the dangers of people who try to solve their weight-loss problem by simply "watching what they eat." He says, "Too many people just cut back on what they eat to an extent that they don't get all of the nutrition that they need and I think many doctors don't recognize what people are doing to themselves. It's the most frustrating thing in medicine, trying to help patients with diet and weight control. Our tools have been so poor. The customary approach is eliminating food instead of paying attention to their basic nutritional requirements. People who self-diet will generally not only avoid the starches, which are relatively unimportant, but also avoid the proteins which make the difference between safety and danger.

"The Micro Diet is unexcelled. It is ideal because it has demonstrated the rapid ability to lower blood sugars, to lower serum cholesterol, to lower elevated blood pressure, and to therapeutically correct the problems that we are trying to deal with in our patients. The Micro Diet program has some attributes which you don't find in other programs—the variety of foods, the ability to provide adequate fiber, the ease of preparation and portability. With this program, dieters are guaranteed total nutritional fulfillment. People stay with this program because they have what they want; they have what they are supposed to have. They have it conveniently and inexpensively, and therefore many more people meet their ultimate goal on this program than any other diet that I've ever seen."

## *DIABETES*

Low-calorie diets are becoming an important treatment option for obese non-insulin-dependent diabetics. Researchers Dr. Jerrold M. Olefsky and Dr. Robert Henry, in a University of California, San Diego, and University of Colorado project, compared a group of obese diabetics and nondiabetics. These patients were taken into a hospital ward and closely monitored for forty days.

Weight loss was rapid, averaging thirty-six pounds per person, and many health benefits were noted. The doctors reported: "excellent acceptance and compliance as well as widespread metabolic benefits.... In the diabetic subjects a variety of metabolic abnormalities resolved, with the attainment of levels comparable to those seen in nondiabetic subjects. The normalization of hyperglycemia (high blood sugar) occurred rapidly, mainly within the first week. Fasting insulin levels also fell rapidly by 50%."

Doctors Olefsky and Henry concluded that the diet demonstrated "excellent efficacy and safety." The obese non-insulin-dependent diabetics, they said, enjoyed "dramatic benefits." The evidence, they felt, was clear that such a weight-loss program "definitely confers an advantage over conventional diet therapy regarding rapidity of weight loss and improvement of metabolic abnormalities."

General practitioner H. Lloyd Alexander, of San Jose, California, is one M.D. who has firsthand experience of the benefits propounded by Doctors Olefsky and Henry. The approach of his forty-fifth high school reunion made him determine to get down to the weight that he had held when he left high school—and that meant dropping thirty-five pounds. He did it in two-and-a-half months and, one year later, having maintained that weight loss, says, "I now have my Type II diabetes under control and I attribute my success to The Micro Diet. As many other dieters report, I cannot believe the energy that I continue to have daily. For the first time in many years I feel good about being in control of my weight. The Micro Diet was fast, easy, completely nutritious, and is now part of my lifestyle. What else could I possibly eat that would provide me with this kind of nutrition?"

Wayne Waggener, a thirty-nine-year-old project engineer of Thurmont, Maryland, was a 330-pound frustrated dieter and a diabetic who says that he nearly lapsed into a coma. Today, after losing ninety pounds, his doctor has taken him off medication. "The Micro Diet has allowed me to have the rapid weight loss, as well as the sound nutrition that I needed to start my 'new' life," he says. "It's the first time that I have ever dieted and felt good. My newfound energy is wonderful. I'm working on projects around the house that I really enjoy but never had the energy to do before. I confuse our four small dogs, because I never sit in my easy chair anymore and they used to climb on my lap for a snooze while I was snoozing."

Wayne's job takes him on the road five days a week and he found it difficult to eat a balanced diet. Now The Micro Diet, as well as a portable gym, travels everywhere with him. Adds Wayne, whose goal is to lose another forty pounds from his 5-foot, 11-inch frame, "My wife loves to hug me now. She can reach all the way round me."

A personal need to lose weight was also the motivating factor for Dr. Bernard Westerling, a clinical professor at the University of Massachusetts Medical School. After shedding thirty-eight pounds in ten weeks, and maintaining that weight loss for two years, he enthusiastically recommends the program to his patients.

"It's one of the most beneficial things I've done in preventive medicine in my career, and I've been practicing for sixteen years now," he says. "From a nutrition point of view The Micro Diet has everything in it that you need. It's very well balanced. You feel healthy, you don't feel hungry or tired, and that's probably because your body is not being deprived of anything. This is a diet for people with a busy lifestyle. There's no weighing or measuring of foods, no cooking. You just add water or eat one of the bars. It is so convenient. In my case I may be working in the intensive care unit in the early hours of the morning and miss a meal. Now I have a quick Micro meal. It keeps me going and I feel good."

Dr. Westerling believes, too, that The Micro Diet support system is very important. "I've been very impressed with the quality of the Micro Diet Advisors. In general, they are a very caring group of people who encourage the dieter every step of the way."

Gulnar Poorsattar, M.D., a lecturer and specialist in endocrinology in Rockford, Illinois, also feels that The Micro Diet is a program whose time has come. "I was very resistant to the idea of a diet based on packaged meals, but when I finally took a serious look I realized that everything you need in a diet has been put together for you. The Micro Diet is really something I have always taught, except that now it comes in a package. People need time to plan a well-balanced meal, but it isn't always easy or practical for them to do so. The Micro Diet does that for them. I recommend the program to patients of all ages. It is not a program that you go 'on' or 'off.' It's a practical program for life, which offers such variety and so many options."

## *TALKING TO YOUR DOCTOR*

We are all unique individuals. We cannot personally monitor you, and you should not assume that because there is so much evidence to support The Micro Diet that it is automatically perfect for you. It is highly recommended that you involve your doctor. Your physician can advise you which of the loser-friendly Micro Diet plans presented in chapters six, seven, and eight is most suitable for you to follow.

## ■ A CASE STUDY
## LINDA PHILLIPS: DANCING FOR JOY

Linda Phillips, who lost 110 pounds, delights in proving the skeptics to be wrong. "Many people are surprised when I tell them how much weight I lost. Most of them don't believe me until I show them my 'before' picture. Then, of course, they want to know how long I've kept it off. Again, they're surprised when I tell them I've maintained my weight loss for close to two years."

A mother of four, Linda, of Lake Helen, Florida, weighed 259 pounds before she found The Micro Diet. She attributes her weight gain, purely and simply, to overeating. "My eating was out of control. I was never hungry. I didn't have the chance to be hungry because I ate all the time."

Linda had tried numerous diets but would always become discouraged with her lack of progress, quit, and gain more weight. "Although I tried many diets, I always really thought I could do it 'my way': no definite plan, still having all the things I liked but less of them. Of course, I didn't want to give up anything, so I never lost much weight. I always thought dieting would be temporary, just until I lost the weight. Then I could go back to eating whatever I wanted. I have finally realized that if I go back to eating like I did before, I will look like I did before. I have finally realized that it is necessary to make permanent changes in my habits. For me, that means continuing to use Micro meals to maintain my weight, but that's no hardship because I really enjoy them. I have become selective now. When I choose to eat something other than a Micro meal, I do not waste calories on junk food. I select a favorite food and slowly savor the taste of it."

The dramatic change in Linda's appearance and lifestyle is vividly illustrated by her experiences at two high school reunions—ten years apart. At the fifteen-year anniversary, she says, "One of the popular boys who used to sit next to me in English asked, 'Were you in my class? I don't remember you.' I'd gained over one hundred pounds. No wonder he didn't recognize me."

It was a different story when Linda, 110 pounds lighter, attended the twenty-fifth reunion and wore a size ten dress instead of an eighteen. When she and her husband arrived at the event, says Linda, she thought they were at the wrong place because everyone looked old to her. "I guess I just feel younger since I've lost so much weight." But the biggest difference of all was displayed when the music began to play.

Says Linda, "In high school there was a group of us that used to hang around together and we'd go to the Y dances and really dance up a storm. One of the guys asked me up to dance and we started to pony, which is very energetic. I was having a good time, dancing away, and he said, 'Linda, you're gonna kill me with this.' He was having a hard time keeping up. When the music ended, he sat down wiping his brow, and I was ready to go again."

Forty-five-year-old Linda now proudly wears a smaller size than she did at her high school graduation and weighs less than at any time in her adult life. "I never ever told my husband how much I weighed. Like, who was I trying to kid? Did I think he didn't know I outweighed him? Now, for the first time since I have known him, I weigh less than he does.

"I have taken charge of my life and The Micro Diet has been the tool I used. I feel good about myself. My self-esteem has soared. The best result I have experienced from this program is the feeling of 'worth' I have received from my family. I always wondered if my children were ashamed of me because I was heavy, or loved me just because I was their mom. I always wondered what my husband saw in me.

"He has always been slim and I've always been proud of him, but I did not fully appreciate it until I lost some weight and noticed how so many men his age are overweight and sloppy-looking. He looks so good. My point is that I now realize how he could have felt all those years being stuck with a fat wife. He has been so supportive and is always telling me how great I look, but if looks were the only basis for love, he would not have been with me for twenty-five years. The Micro Diet is the tool I used to find this out for myself. It's a catalyst to help people realize that they are the kind of person they have always wanted to be, but did not have the confidence to see in themselves.

"Through the Micro Diet I have learned that I do not have to deprive myself of everything I like for the rest of my life. Who could do that? Forever is a long time. Now I know what to eat most of the time, when to eat it, and when I can have something that may not be very good for me. I also know I cannot do this all the time but I have learned not to feel guilty, abnormal, and dump the whole diet because of one error. The Micro Diet is forgiving. If I cheat today, I can start right back on the diet tomorrow and still keep losing. My weight loss may slow down, but I am still making progress."

For Linda, one of the greatest assets of The Micro Diet program is her Advisor, Suzanne de Rham. They met at a home show when Suzanne gave her a sample meal and an invitation to attend a meeting. Linda, skeptical about "yet another" diet program, reluctantly attended. Three years later, they still get together every week or so to "keep tabs on each other" by discussing their progress and providing encouragement when needed.

# 5

# THE SURVEY OF SUCCESS

RAPID WEIGHT LOSS. Permanent weight maintenance. Specific health improvements. Over the years we have heard countless tremendously exciting success stories. Quantifying that success, however, was not possible until the University of Surrey's Dr. Stordy undertook a succession of nationwide surveys in Great Britain.

Initially, Dr. Stordy randomly distributed an extensive questionnaire to a number of Micro Diet Advisors. The Advisors, in turn, handed the questionnaire to every third client commencing their third (or more) week on the diet. The clients then returned the completed questionnaires directly to Dr. Stordy. There were 855 respondents (88.5% women; average age forty-one) producing some highly illuminating results.

A total of 67% said that they had discovered The Micro Diet through the word-of-mouth recommendation of a relative, friend, or acquaintance while 5.4% had been encouraged to use the diet by a health professional. Not surprisingly (since many dieters pursue numerous diets during the course of a lifetime), 95% of those surveyed said that they had previously tried other methods of losing weight. The majority had simply cut calories while 38% had invested money in commercial weight-loss establishments.

### *AN AMAZING 94% FOUND IT EASIER TO LOSE WEIGHT WITH THE MICRO DIET THAN OTHER METHODS.*

Quite importantly, the dieter's family turned out to be more supportive of their weight loss efforts with The Micro Diet program than with other methods—75% as opposed to 53%, actually provided "active encouragement." The reason for this was not elicited in the survey, but it certainly will confound critics who believe a low-calorie plan to be socially disruptive. I can only assume that the dieter was enjoying success, becoming happier, and as a result the family rallied round in support.

The role of the Micro Diet Advisor is to give support and encouragement and we were delighted to note that 77% of the survey group felt that the role of the Advisor had been either "very important" or "fairly important" in helping them achieve their weight loss. Most of the respondents were still on the weight loss path and incredibly motivated, since 96.4% said that they believed they would reach their target through The Micro Diet. Those dieters who had already achieved their goal (31%) were asked the all-important question about keeping the weight off.

## *86% FOUND IT WAS "EASY" OR "EASIER" TO MAINTAIN THEIR TARGET WEIGHT WITH THE MICRO DIET.*

A total of 89% of the respondents were continuing to use Micro meals as an implicit part of their weight maintenance program, while 76.7% said that their dietary habits had changed since starting the program. This statistic is particularly significant as one of the primary criticisms of low-calorie diets is "they don't teach long-term eating habits." But with The Micro Diet this isn't true. The program incorporates lifestyle choices for lifetime weight maintenance. It is not just a rapid weight-loss plan.

Says Kevin Nahm, M.D., of Newberg, Oregon, who with his wife, Alice, has lost a combined total of forty-five pounds, "A side benefit for us is that our fifteen-year-old daughter, just by watching us, is picking up better eating habits. At her age, of course, she isn't dieting but she is following our example and definitely being more selective in what she eats. This has had a very positive impact on our family."

Adds Dr. Nahm, who specializes in obstetrics and gynecology, "Many of my patients are heavy and, until now, I felt I couldn't do anything for them. As for my own wife, this is the first time in her life that she has been able to lose weight. The Micro Diet is convenient and it really works."

That's the kind of positive reaction to the program that we are hearing more and more from members of the medical community, and, in fact, the University of Surrey survey also revealed that:

### *71% OF THOSE DOCTORS CONSULTED BY THE DIETERS "ACTIVELY ENCOURAGED" WEIGHT LOSS WITH THE MICRO DIET.*

Anyone wishing to start the diet should check with a doctor first so that he or she can monitor progress and form a firsthand appreciation of the benefits of the program. During the course of the weight-loss regimen, the vast majority of dieters, 97.2%, had no need at all to consult their doctors with any problems. A small number of dieters experienced minor temporary complaints (most easily remedied by drinking more water) such as headaches, constipation, dizziness, bad breath, and hunger. The vast majority, however, commented on improvements in their sense of well-being.

### *89% "FELT WELL" ON THE DIET, 71% NOTICED HEALTH IMPROVEMENT.*

Says Dr. Stordy, "The results from the survey were very impressive. It is obvious that a great many people have clearly benefitted from their experience with The Micro Diet."

A second follow-up survey, also conducted at the University of Surrey, produced some even more impressive statistics. When 112 of the participants in the original study were contacted two-and-a-half years later, 33% of them maintained that they had not regained a single pound. That's a tremendous success rate.

Even those dieters who had regained some weight were still 40% to 50% lighter than they had been before the diet, and the entire group's mean Body Mass Index (a way of categorizing the extent of obesity, explained in Chapter Six) had significantly moved down from the obese to the overweight classification, putting them at considerably less health risk.

Of those respondents who still needed to lose weight, 71.7% said they would use The Micro Diet to achieve their goal, a clear indication that they were happy with the program and felt no need to look elsewhere for the solution to their weight problem.

Over two-thirds of this sample also said that they had changed their dietary habits to help maintain their weight. A total of 62.5% indicated that they now consciously choose low-calorie alternatives while 75% and 71.4% had made a deliberate reduction in their intake of sugar and fat respectively. Thirty-nine point three percent of subjects said that they now stop eating when they are no longer hungry, and 55.4% eat only at planned meal times. Forty-three point eight percent claimed a greater appreciation of food.

Asked about their overall feelings toward The Micro Diet program, only 1.8% expressed disappointment, and 72.3% saw themselves continuing to use the meals for weight maintenance.

## ■ A CASE STUDY

### PEGGY OLDS: A "FEEL GOOD" BINGE

"I can eat anyone under the table." That used to be the "proud" boast of self-confessed foodaholic Peggy Olds. "I was a compulsive eater," says Peggy. "I would eat untold amounts of food. Before The Micro Diet, I had never gone three weeks in my life without binge-eating. I've always had this problem and, like an alcoholic I know I always will, but now I can control it. I would much rather have a Micro bar than a candy bar."

A typical lunch for Peggy, a tax accountant from Bay City, Texas, used to be six pieces of her favorite fried chicken, a pint of coleslaw, and a pint of mashed potatoes. She would normally eat three helpings of everything. When she went out for a hamburger, she would go to three different restaurants and order a double cheeseburger at each so that no one would realize how much she was eating. At the grocery store she would often pick up three half-pound chocolate bars. If she got a funny look from the checkout clerk she would explain "I have lots of baking to do." Says Peggy, "You learn to be sneaky and secretive when you eat the amount of food I did."

With that kind of lifestyle, it was not surprising that Peggy ballooned to 285 pounds after losing and regaining hundreds of pounds over the years. She had accepted the fact that she would probably get heavier and heavier. Then she was introduced to The Micro Diet and decided to go for it. In the first ten days she shed ten pounds. She lost thirty-two pounds in two months and, in just over a year, got rid of 135 pounds. In the process, fifty-six-year-old Peggy went from a 46–43–46 figure to 35–29–36, a shape she has maintained for more than a year.

Says Peggy, "I have not binged since I've been on The Micro Diet. I think that if people make an initial three-week commitment to The Micro Diet, it will change their life forever. When people ask me how The Micro Diet differs from other programs, I tell them it's the way it makes you feel. I've never felt so good. Now that I've solved the biggest problem of my life, there are so many things that I want to do. It is truly a new life. It's not only the energy I have, it's the sense of accomplishment which gives you such confidence. I know that this time it will be for the rest of my life. What a statement to be able to make. I am such a food addict that I feel if it can work for me, it can work for anyone. It's so wonderful to be able to recommend a truly safe program that's going to improve your health."

Peggy attributes her success in maintaining the weight loss to learning new eating habits through the Micro Diet program. "I don't want fried food anymore. I honestly thought I couldn't live without it. Now I'm repulsed by the sight and smell of anything fried. I've also lost my cravings for sweets. I have three Micro meals every day to ensure I get solid nutrition and, of course, I incorporate other foods and have learned to cut out the 'extras.' When people ask me if I'm going to stay on this for the rest of my life, I tell them that I'm eating healthier than I have ever done before, so why not?"

Exercise is also now a part of Peggy's lifestyle. "I would hardly walk more than a few steps. That's how physically inactive and out-of-shape I was. It had been seventeen years since I'd done anything really active. I now do it because I enjoy it. I walk two miles nearly every day. I started out slowly, walking just once around the neighborhood high school track. Gradually, I built up to walking four times around it, which equalled a mile. Several months later I achieved the two-mile mark. What a change in my life."

# 6
# GETTING STARTED

GO TO A FULL-LENGTH MIRROR and take a long, hard look at yourself. Do you like what you see? If you see unshapely, unwanted fat spoiling how you look and feel, and you're willing to take control of your life and change it, congratulations. You've just taken another positive move toward a trimmer body. Just imagine what it will be like to lose those extra pounds, to be lighter on your feet, to be able to wear stylish clothes, to look and feel healthier. Here's how you get started.

## *CONSULT YOUR DOCTOR*

Your first step, as with any diet, is to visit your doctor so that your initial state of health can be determined. Make sure you establish your starting weight, blood pressure, and cholesterol levels. Show this book to your physician and point out the excellent nutritional profile of the meals and the medical references section at the end. Discuss the respective merits of using the program as your exclusive source of nutrition (three or four Micro meals a day), or for two meals a day along with another low-fat meal (full details are contained in this chapter).

## *TAKE A PICTURE*

Before you begin the diet, have a good picture taken of yourself. Like many others you may shy away from cameras when you weigh more, but once you've slimmed down you'll want a "before" photograph to proudly compare the difference, and as a constant reminder not to slip back. Why not have a photograph taken every month to record your progress? Make a point of noticing specific improvements in the shape of your body, and congratulate yourself.

## *HOW MUCH DO YOU NEED TO LOSE?*

Before commencing the diet you must have a clear idea of your goal. It's not good enough to say "I want to get rid of twenty or thirty pounds," or "I'll just see how it goes." A specific target is essential. So how much do you need to lose? Quite probably you've checked your status before with the "weight for height" chart published by the Metropolitan Life Insurance Company. A more accurate guideline can be ascertained with a method most health professionals are now using: the Body Mass Index or BMI. To discover your BMI you take your weight in kilos and divide it by your height in meters squared.

Sounds complicated? Don't worry, the accompanying chart has already done the mathematics for you. Simply cross-check your weight and height and you'll find your BMI. The latest information, from leading researchers, is that the desirable Body Mass Index for men and women should be adjusted according to age. For 19–34-year-olds, the BMI range should be 20–25; age 35–44, BMI 21–26; age 45–54, BMI 22–27; age 55–64, BMI 23–28; and age 65 plus, BMI 24–29.

## *WEIGH IN*

Accurately weigh yourself and make sure that throughout your diet plan you weigh yourself first thing in the morning wearing the same clothes (or none at all).

## *MORALE-BOOSTER*

Find a way of recording your progress. Some dieters like to fill a box with heavy objects to represent that excess weight—books or stones, for instance. As the pounds disappear, they remove the corresponding weight in objects. It's wonderfully encouraging to find yourself physically "throwing away the fat." If this is too time-consuming or the box takes up too much space,

# BODY MASS INDEX CHART

| height (in.) | 60 | 61 | 62 | 63 | 64 | 65 | 66 | 67 | 68 | 69 | 70 | 71 | 72 | 73 |
|---|---|---|---|---|---|---|---|---|---|---|---|---|---|---|
| height (ft.-in.) | 5′0″ | 5′1″ | 5′2″ | 5′3″ | 5′4″ | 5′5″ | 5′6″ | 5′7″ | 5′8″ | 5′9″ | 5′10″ | 5′11″ | 6′0″ | 6′1″ |
| weight (lbs.) | Follow your weight in pounds to your height and read your Body Mass Index | | | | | | | | | | | | | |
| 100 | 19.5 | 18.9 | 18.3 | 17.7 | 17.2 | 16.7 | 16.2 | 15.7 | 15.2 | 14.8 | 14.4 | 14.0 | 13.6 | 13.2 |
| 105 | 20.5 | 19.9 | 19.2 | 18.6 | 18.0 | 17.5 | 17.0 | 16.5 | 16.0 | 15.5 | 15.1 | 14.7 | 14.3 | 13.9 |
| 110 | 21.5 | 20.8 | 20.1 | 19.5 | 18.9 | 18.3 | 17.8 | 17.2 | 16.7 | 16.3 | 15.8 | 15.4 | 14.9 | 14.5 |
| 115 | 22.5 | 21.7 | 21.1 | 20.4 | 19.8 | 19.2 | 18.6 | 18.0 | 17.5 | 17.0 | 16.5 | 16.1 | 15.6 | 15.2 |
| 120 | 23.5 | 22.7 | 22.0 | 21.3 | 20.6 | 20.0 | 19.4 | 18.8 | 18.3 | 17.7 | 17.2 | 16.8 | 16.3 | 15.8 |
| 125 | 24.4 | 23.6 | 22.9 | 22.2 | 21.5 | 20.8 | 20.2 | 19.6 | 19.0 | 18.5 | 18.0 | 17.4 | 17.0 | 16.5 |
| 130 | 25.4 | 24.6 | 23.8 | 23.0 | 22.3 | 21.7 | 21.0 | 20.4 | 19.8 | 19.2 | 18.7 | 18.1 | 17.6 | 17.2 |
| 135 | 26.4 | 25.5 | 24.7 | 23.9 | 23.2 | 22.5 | 21.8 | 21.2 | 20.5 | 20.0 | 19.4 | 18.8 | 18.3 | 17.8 |
| 140 | 27.4 | 26.5 | 25.6 | 24.8 | 24.1 | 23.3 | 22.6 | 21.9 | 21.3 | 20.7 | 20.1 | 19.5 | 19.0 | 18.5 |
| 145 | 28.3 | 27.4 | 26.5 | 25.7 | 24.9 | 24.2 | 23.4 | 22.7 | 22.1 | 21.4 | 20.8 | 20.2 | 19.7 | 19.1 |
| 150 | 29.3 | 28.4 | 27.5 | 26.6 | 25.8 | 25.0 | 24.2 | 23.5 | 22.8 | 22.2 | 21.5 | 20.9 | 20.4 | 19.8 |
| 155 | 30.3 | 29.3 | 28.4 | 27.5 | 26.6 | 25.8 | 25.0 | 24.3 | 23.6 | 22.9 | 22.3 | 21.6 | 21.0 | 20.5 |
| 160 | 31.3 | 30.3 | 29.3 | 28.4 | 27.5 | 26.6 | 25.8 | 25.1 | 24.3 | 23.6 | 23.0 | 22.3 | 21.7 | 21.1 |
| 165 | 32.3 | 31.2 | 30.2 | 29.3 | 28.3 | 27.5 | 26.7 | 25.9 | 25.1 | 24.4 | 23.7 | 23.0 | 22.4 | 21.8 |
| 170 | 33.2 | 32.1 | 31.1 | 30.1 | 29.2 | 28.3 | 27.5 | 26.6 | 25.9 | 25.1 | 24.4 | 23.7 | 23.1 | 22.4 |
| 175 | 34.2 | 33.1 | 32.0 | 31.0 | 30.1 | 29.1 | 28.3 | 27.4 | 26.6 | 25.9 | 25.1 | 24.4 | 23.8 | 23.1 |
| 180 | 35.2 | 34.0 | 33.0 | 31.9 | 30.9 | 30.0 | 29.1 | 28.2 | 27.4 | 26.6 | 25.9 | 25.1 | 24.4 | 23.8 |
| 185 | 36.2 | 35.0 | 33.9 | 32.8 | 31.8 | 30.8 | 29.9 | 29.0 | 28.2 | 27.3 | 26.6 | 25.8 | 25.1 | 24.4 |
| 190 | 37.1 | 35.9 | 34.8 | 33.7 | 32.6 | 31.6 | 30.7 | 29.8 | 28.9 | 28.1 | 27.3 | 26.5 | 25.8 | 25.1 |
| 195 | 38.1 | 36.9 | 35.7 | 34.6 | 33.5 | 32.5 | 31.5 | 30.6 | 29.7 | 28.8 | 28.0 | 27.2 | 26.5 | 25.8 |
| 200 | 39.1 | 37.8 | 36.6 | 35.5 | 34.4 | 33.3 | 32.3 | 31.4 | 30.4 | 29.6 | 28.7 | 27.9 | 27.1 | 26.4 |
| 205 | 40.1 | 38.8 | 37.5 | 36.3 | 35.2 | 34.1 | 33.1 | 32.1 | 31.2 | 30.3 | 29.4 | 28.6 | 27.8 | 27.1 |
| 210 | 41.0 | 39.7 | 38.4 | 37.2 | 36.1 | 35.0 | 33.9 | 32.9 | 32.0 | 31.0 | 30.2 | 29.3 | 28.5 | 27.7 |
| 215 | 42.0 | 40.7 | 39.4 | 38.1 | 36.9 | 35.8 | 34.7 | 33.7 | 32.7 | 31.8 | 30.9 | 30.0 | 29.2 | 28.4 |

| | | | | | | | | | | | | | | |
|---|---|---|---|---|---|---|---|---|---|---|---|---|---|---|
| 220 | 43.0 | 41.6 | 40.3 | 39.0 | 37.8 | 36.6 | 35.5 | 34.5 | 33.5 | 32.5 | 31.6 | 30.7 | 29.9 | 29.1 |
| 225 | 44.0 | 42.6 | 41.2 | 39.9 | 38.7 | 37.5 | 36.3 | 35.3 | 34.2 | 33.3 | 32.3 | 31.4 | 30.5 | 29.7 |
| 230 | 45.0 | 43.5 | 42.1 | 40.8 | 39.5 | 38.3 | 37.2 | 36.1 | 35.0 | 34.0 | 33.0 | 32.1 | 31.2 | 30.4 |
| 235 | 45.9 | 44.4 | 43.0 | 41.7 | 40.4 | 39.1 | 38.0 | 36.8 | 35.8 | 34.7 | 33.7 | 32.8 | 31.9 | 31.0 |
| 240 | 46.9 | 45.4 | 43.9 | 42.6 | 41.2 | 40.0 | 38.8 | 37.6 | 36.5 | 35.5 | 34.5 | 33.5 | 32.6 | 31.7 |
| 245 | 47.9 | 46.3 | 44.9 | 43.4 | 42.1 | 40.8 | 39.6 | 38.4 | 37.3 | 36.2 | 35.2 | 34.2 | 33.3 | 32.4 |
| 250 | 48.9 | 47.3 | 45.8 | 44.3 | 43.0 | 41.6 | 40.4 | 39.2 | 38.0 | 37.0 | 35.9 | 34.9 | 33.9 | 33.0 |
| 255 | 49.8 | 48.2 | 46.7 | 45.2 | 43.8 | 42.5 | 41.2 | 40.0 | 38.8 | 37.7 | 36.6 | 35.6 | 34.6 | 33.7 |
| 260 | 50.8 | 49.2 | 47.6 | 46.1 | 44.7 | 43.3 | 42.0 | 40.8 | 39.6 | 38.4 | 37.3 | 36.3 | 35.3 | 34.3 |
| 265 | 51.8 | 50.1 | 48.5 | 47.0 | 45.5 | 44.1 | 42.8 | 41.5 | 40.3 | 39.2 | 38.1 | 37.0 | 36.0 | 35.0 |
| 270 | 52.8 | 51.1 | 49.4 | 47.9 | 46.4 | 45.0 | 43.6 | 42.3 | 41.1 | 39.9 | 38.8 | 37.7 | 36.7 | 35.7 |
| 275 | 53.8 | 52.0 | 50.3 | 48.8 | 47.2 | 45.8 | 44.4 | 43.1 | 41.9 | 40.6 | 39.5 | 38.4 | 37.3 | 36.3 |
| 280 | 54.7 | 53.0 | 51.3 | 49.6 | 48.1 | 46.6 | 45.2 | 43.9 | 42.6 | 41.4 | 40.2 | 39.1 | 38.0 | 37.0 |
| 285 | 55.7 | 53.9 | 52.2 | 50.5 | 49.0 | 47.5 | 46.0 | 44.7 | 43.4 | 42.1 | 40.9 | 39.8 | 38.7 | 37.6 |
| 290 | 56.7 | 54.8 | 53.1 | 51.4 | 49.8 | 48.3 | 46.8 | 45.5 | 44.1 | 42.9 | 41.6 | 40.5 | 39.4 | 38.3 |
| 295 | 57.7 | 55.8 | 54.0 | 52.3 | 50.7 | 49.1 | 47.7 | 46.2 | 44.9 | 43.6 | 42.4 | 41.2 | 40.0 | 39.0 |
| 300 | 58.6 | 56.7 | 54.9 | 53.2 | 51.5 | 50.0 | 48.5 | 47.0 | 45.7 | 44.3 | 43.1 | 41.9 | 40.7 | 39.6 |
| 305 | 59.6 | 57.7 | 55.8 | 54.1 | 52.4 | 50.8 | 49.3 | 47.8 | 46.4 | 45.1 | 43.8 | 42.6 | 41.4 | 40.3 |
| 310 | 60.6 | 58.6 | 56.8 | 55.0 | 53.3 | 51.6 | 50.1 | 48.6 | 47.2 | 45.8 | 44.5 | 43.3 | 42.1 | 40.9 |
| 315 | 61.6 | 59.6 | 57.7 | 55.8 | 54.1 | 52.5 | 50.9 | 49.4 | 47.9 | 46.6 | 45.2 | 44.0 | 42.8 | 41.6 |
| 320 | 62.6 | 60.5 | 58.6 | 56.7 | 55.0 | 53.3 | 51.7 | 50.2 | 48.7 | 47.3 | 46.0 | 44.7 | 43.4 | 42.3 |
| 325 | 63.5 | 61.5 | 59.5 | 57.6 | 55.8 | 54.1 | 52.5 | 50.9 | 49.5 | 48.0 | 46.7 | 45.4 | 44.1 | 42.9 |
| 330 | 64.5 | 62.4 | 60.4 | 58.5 | 56.7 | 55.0 | 53.3 | 51.7 | 50.2 | 48.8 | 47.4 | 46.1 | 44.8 | 43.6 |
| 335 | 65.5 | 63.4 | 61.3 | 59.4 | 57.6 | 55.8 | 54.1 | 52.5 | 51.0 | 49.5 | 48.1 | 46.8 | 45.5 | 44.2 |
| 340 | 66.5 | 64.3 | 62.2 | 60.3 | 58.4 | 56.6 | 54.9 | 53.3 | 51.7 | 50.3 | 48.8 | 47.5 | 46.2 | 44.9 |
| 345 | 67.4 | 65.2 | 63.2 | 61.2 | 59.3 | 57.5 | 55.7 | 54.1 | 52.5 | 51.0 | 49.5 | 48.2 | 46.8 | 45.6 |
| 350 | 68.4 | 66.2 | 64.1 | 62.1 | 60.1 | 58.3 | 56.5 | 54.9 | 53.3 | 51.7 | 50.3 | 48.9 | 47.5 | 46.2 |
| 355 | 69.4 | 67.1 | 65.0 | 62.9 | 61.0 | 59.1 | 57.3 | 55.7 | 54.0 | 52.5 | 51.0 | 49.6 | 48.2 | 46.9 |
| 360 | 70.4 | 68.1 | 65.9 | 63.8 | 61.8 | 60.0 | 58.2 | 56.4 | 54.8 | 53.2 | 51.7 | 50.3 | 48.9 | 47.5 |
| 365 | 71.3 | 69.0 | 66.8 | 64.7 | 62.7 | 60.8 | 59.0 | 57.2 | 55.5 | 53.9 | 52.4 | 51.0 | 49.5 | 48.2 |
| 370 | 72.3 | 70.0 | 67.7 | 65.6 | 63.6 | 61.6 | 59.8 | 58.0 | 56.3 | 54.7 | 53.1 | 51.7 | 50.2 | 48.9 |
| 375 | 73.3 | 70.9 | 68.6 | 66.5 | 64.4 | 62.5 | 60.6 | 58.8 | 57.1 | 55.4 | 53.9 | 52.3 | 50.9 | 49.5 |
| 380 | 74.3 | 71.9 | 69.6 | 67.4 | 65.3 | 63.3 | 61.4 | 59.6 | 57.8 | 56.2 | 54.6 | 53.0 | 51.6 | 50.2 |
| 385 | 75.3 | 72.8 | 70.5 | 68.3 | 66.1 | 64.1 | 62.2 | 60.4 | 58.6 | 56.9 | 55.3 | 53.7 | 52.3 | 50.8 |
| 390 | 76.2 | 73.8 | 71.4 | 69.1 | 67.0 | 65.0 | 63.0 | 61.1 | 59.4 | 57.6 | 56.0 | 54.4 | 52.9 | 51.5 |

you could set two glass jars near the bathroom scales. Place marbles into one jar (each marble counting as one of your unwanted pounds) and transfer the marbles according to your weight loss. It will be an extremely positive morale booster.

One person who followed this advice ended up transferring the grand total of 135 marbles in just fourteen months. "Muff" Juber, a 58-year-old grandmother of fourteen, was justifiably proud of her collection and, two years later, her jar still holds 135 marbles. During the two-year period of weight maintenance she says, she never had to transfer more than five marbles out of the "success" jar, because she never regained more than five pounds.

"Muff," of Renton, Washington, says, "I used to eat without paying attention to the nutritional value of what I snacked on. I just ate without thinking. The marbles kept me on track. They made me concentrate on what I was doing."

When she began the diet, Muff took two quart-size glass jars, placed them next to each other on her kitchen windowsill, and filled one with 135 marbles (including two large ones). Initially, she found that looking at those jars was "daunting," but she got over that hurdle by setting herself a short-term goal of transferring enough marbles to cover the bottom of the empty jar. She celebrated each ten pounds of progress by transferring a brightly colored marble. At the fifty and 100 pound milestones she transferred the larger marbles.

Says Muff, "It kept my weight-loss goal in front of my eyes so I never lost sight of it. Even today the two jars remain on my windowsill as a constant reminder of what I have achieved. I feel great. I feel like a recycled teenager."

Executive chef Bill McLeish, of Doraville, Georgia, took a slightly more dramatic approach. "For every five pounds I lost, I put a five-pound brick in my suitcase. Can you imagine carrying around eighty extra pounds like that? It really made me appreciate just how heavy I had gotten."

## *DIETING MADE EASY*

Flexibility and simplicity are two important "loser-friendly" words. *Flexibility* means you have the opportunity to choose a program to suit your individual lifestyle. I don't feel it is at all appropriate to lay down rigid guidelines and insist that everyone obey them. I don't see the point in becoming a martyr to a diet regimen, or suffering excruciating pangs of guilt because you "sneaked" a chocolate cookie. Micro meals are so low in calories, a few extra calories are not going to be disastrous. You may not lose weight that day, but you'll probably not gain weight. That's why I regard the loser-friendly Micro Diet as the benevolent diet.

*Simplicity* means that the guesswork is taken out of dieting. Perfect nutrition in so few calories makes The Micro Diet a sophisticated diet; yet following the 800–1,000-calorie "sole source" plan couldn't be easier. There are no calories to count. No foods to weigh. No portions to control. No complicated food exchanges to makes. You don't have to search the supermarkets for exotic fruits and vegetables, and you don't have to spend hours laboring in the kitchen. You can if you want to, but the choice is yours. All the work has been done for you.

## *THE CHOICE IS YOURS*

There's a weight-loss plan to suit everyone—because you get to choose the way you want to use The Micro Diet. We are all unique. We have different lifestyles. What works for me may not work for you. But the loser-friendly Micro Diet works for everyone...everyone, that is, who wants it to work. It works because there are so many options that the program never becomes boring. Here are some of the choices:

### 1. The 800–1,000-Calorie "Sole Source" Plan.

The simplest, fastest way to lose weight is by eating three or four Micro meals a day, and nothing else except plenty of liquids, preferably eight glasses of water (and some raw vegetables, if you like). You will be able to select from a wide array of appetizing meals, including entrees such as chicken tetrazzini, chili, and Spanish rice; breakfast cereals including muesli; satisfying, filling bars such as peanut, yogurt-orange, muesli, chocolate—even popcorn; chocolate, vanilla, and strawberry shakes; and tomato, pea, and chicken soups.

This plan provides complete, balanced nutrition in a recommended minimum of 800 calories a day. The great advantage of this method is that, without any effort on your part, you know exactly how many calories you are consuming. You know your body is being fed a superb balance of all of the nutrients that you need. It also removes many of the everyday temptations that you encounter on other diets such as grocery shopping, preparing the food, and cooking the meal. It's so easy, isn't it, to allow yourself a "small" extra portion, or "forget yourself," and just have a "little taste" when you're doling out the portions? Before long your 1,000-calorie plan has had several hundred extra calories added to it, which somehow go uncounted.

Isn't an 800-calorie level too low? Absolutely not. Remember, it's not the calories that count, it's the nutritional quality of those calories. You already have those extra calories stored on your body as fat. Today's very low-calorie diets and low-calorie diets, in general, have been designed to ensure that you receive all of the protein and other essential nutrients to keep your body healthy while losing weight. There is now overwhelming scientific and public experience to support this level of calorie intake and many scientists, in fact, prefer that the dieter embark on this course of action. The fast weight loss is so motivating that you will find it easier to stick to the diet and achieve your goal.

But for how long? Clinical trials with diets at the much lower levels of 330 and 420 calories a day, have positively shown that dieters with a real need to lose weight (in excess of thirty pounds) can use such programs for extended periods of time, certainly several months.

Even though three to four meals provides at least 800 calories a day, we strongly recommend that you use the Micro meals as your only source of food for a maximum of three weeks at a time followed by a fourth week in which another low-calorie meal is eaten in addition to, or instead of, one Micro meal. This will help you practice incorporating a variety of foods into your diet during that fourth week. In the everyday world you will be called upon to make eating choices in the home and outside. The sooner you begin to make small, easy changes, the sooner you will be able to adopt a lifestyle which will keep you trim and healthy. (Micro meals make it easy to lose weight on this "sole source" plan, but you'll soon discover how they also form part of an ongoing healthier-eating plan.)

As long as you have fat stores to burn, this three-week–one-week pattern can be observed until you reach your target weight.

Tom Johnston, of the U.S. Virgin Islands, made a wholehearted "sole source" commitment and got rid of 115 pounds.

"It was easier for me to go "sole source" without facing the temptation of ice-cream or other foods. I felt great doing it that way."

Sixty-one-year-old Tom has maintained his weight loss for four years—in spite of the fact that he owns a pizza restaurant. "I cook and bake at the restaurant, but I know I'll never put the weight back on because I've learned how to avoid fats. I know extremely well how much fat and how many calories go into my pizzas!" Adds Tom, "I've become more physically and socially active. My life has changed completely. People who have known me for years have failed to recognize me."

Does a three-week commitment to eating nothing but Micro meals sound like a long time? Then, give it five. Not five weeks, just five days. Make a five-day commitment to use the program and nothing else. You have probably spent a lifetime gaining the extra weight, so don't you owe it to yourself to make a five-day effort to lose it? The initial weight loss and feeling of well-being can be so exciting that you will be motivated to continue with the plan.

That's what happened to Donna Sheposh, of Spokane, Washington. "I committed myself to five days only," she says. "Those five days were so exciting I committed to two weeks. In those two weeks I lost twenty pounds and dropped two dress sizes. At the end of five months I had lost seventy-six pounds, felt dynamic, looked terrific and was being courted by a delightful, handsome gentleman who was a youth worker at my church. He had never taken that kind of interest in me before."

That courtship led to marriage, says forty-year-old Donna, who, two-and-a-half years later, has kept every pound off. Donna, who had been overweight for eighteen years before The Micro Diet entered her life, says, "You can quit smoking. You can be cured of drugs. But you can't quit eating, and eating was my addiction. I would eat for comfort, for pleasure, or because I was stressed-out. I believe I succeeded because of the healthy nature of these meals. The Micro Diet set me free from the bondage of food. It was a way for me to separate myself from other food long enough so I could break years of bad habits. After my second day on the diet, I felt energetic and really good. I've eaten one or two, sometimes three, Micro meals a day ever since. It's a safety guard for me."

Carole Culp, of Spokane, Washington, also quickly became

convinced that the program would work for her. "I knew after just one week that the diet would work. I liked the taste, my hunger was minimal, and my energy level was improving. It was so easy." Carole, who has maintained her goal weight for over two years, says that she gained forty pounds after she quit smoking. Her doctor's advice was to simply "eat less, exercise more." She tried to do that, but to no avail. Then she was introduced to The Micro Diet.

"My health is so improved now. I feel better than I have in years, and my self-esteem is at an all-time high," says forty-six-year-old Carole, who also sings the praises of the Advisor support system. "The Advisors in my area have been true friends. They are truly a very special breed of caring people." Adds Carole, "The Micro Diet has changed my life. It just cannot be surpassed for weight loss, good nutrition, and weight maintenance. By the time a person loses weight with the program they find that they have retrained their habits to include healthy choices."

### 2. "Sole Source"/Fiber Plus.

Eat your three or four Micro meals and add some high-fiber foods such as fruits and vegetables. Weight loss will still be rapid. You will satisfy the need to crunch, you will practice adding other highly nutritious foods to your diet, and you certainly won't be hungry.

### 3. The 1,000–1,200-Calorie Plan.

Keep your choice-making easy by selecting two Micro meals and preparing one other low-fat "enhanced" Micro meal (through adding other nourishing foods). Alternatively, you could elect to embark on a "Two Plus One" regimen—two Micro meals plus one "other" low-calorie meal. Weight loss may be slower (depending on your choice of food, you may find that you slip above the 1,200-calorie level). This plan does, of course, give you the flexibility of eating one meal with family or friends. If your weight loss is too slow—or screeches to a halt—cut back on the amount in your added meal. I recommend you have the "regular" meal for breakfast or lunch rather than in the evening, as your intake is likely to be more modest at these times.

Thirty-seven-year-old Mita del Fierro followed the Two Plus One program and lost forty pounds in ten weeks. "It was so easy," she says. "I was totally satisfied and I lost my craving for sweets and snacks, which had been my big problem."

Mita, of Seattle, Washington, had never had a weight problem in her life until she gained seventy-five pounds with her first pregnancy. She subsequently managed to lose all but ten to fifteen pounds, but with her second child gained another fifty-five. Most of that stayed put. "Being heavy wasn't a natural thing for me," she remembers. "I saw myself as thin, even though I was heavy. I simply denied that I was overweight. The more weight I gained, I just bought bigger and bigger clothes; clothes with elastic waistbands and loose clothing so that no one could tell where my body began and where my body ended. I hid my figure for the longest time. One day my eyes were opened when I bent down to pick up a mirror on the floor and really saw myself. I noticed the rolls of fat on my neck and thought, 'This is me?' The image in the mirror didn't reflect my internal image of myself. I was disgusted with myself and said, 'This has got to stop.'"

A friend recommended The Micro Diet. When she lost eight pounds in the first week, Mita knew it was going to work. At five-foot, three-inches, and weighing 162 pounds, she was "a tight size fourteen." After losing the forty pounds she celebrated by going to buy a new dress, anticipating she would slip into a size ten. "When I tried on those tens they were big. My heart started pounding. I'm saying to myself, 'Can this be true?' And I had the sales gal go and get some eights and some of those were fitting loose and I thought, this can't be. So, I told her to get me some size sixes because I didn't want a situation where I was in a size six just from one particular manufacturer. When I got into all of those sixes, I was jumping up and down and literally shrieking. The sales gal came running in wanting to know what was wrong. I was so excited. It made me realize, there and then, that I had found the real me."

Mita maintains her new figure by having at least one Micro meal a day "out of convenience and habit" and walking at least three times a week.

### 4. The Combo.

Follow the 800–1,000-calorie "sole source" plan during the week (three or four Micro meals a day) and at the weekend go on the 1,000–1,200-calorie plan. Instead of one of the Micro meals, take the "Two Plus One" route and go out for a lunch, or cook yourself something special (and healthy). This approach gives you the opportunity to fully enjoy social occasions without feeling deprived.

### 5. The Alternator.

You could also alternate days—"sole source" one day, "Two Plus One" the next. Again, it is important to bear in mind that the rate of weight loss will vary and that you have to consider what is most suitable for your life.

### 6. Take Your Pick.

"Sole source" or "Two Plus One"? A three-week commitment or a five-day commitment? Weekdays "on" and weekends "off," or one day "on" and one day "off"? It's really up to you. You need to balance the amount of weight you wish to lose and the rate of weight loss you desire with the changes you are prepared to make in your current lifestyle. The choice is yours.

## *THE MICRO DIET OPTIONS*

Don't make the mistake of thinking that a low-calorie plan must be boring or like "taking medicine." Far from it! The loser-friendly Micro Diet program has been designed to satisfy your taste buds any hour of the day and new meals are constantly being added to your range of choices.

Says Muff Juber, "I believe the single most important way to lose and maintain weight is to vary the meals. My husband and I are always trying new recipes that will aid us in eating smarter."

## *MEALS IN A MOMENT*

To be able to fix delicious Micro Diet meals you don't have to be an executive chef like Bill McLeish (who you'll meet in Chapter 8). You just couldn't ask for anything more convenient, as each meal is individually packaged for you. The extent of the demand on your culinary skills is mixing some of the products with water, and stirring.

That was the major attraction for sixty-nine-year-old bachelor John Kanary, of Tampa, Florida, who says, "I don't really cook, so the foods are very convenient for me." John, who lost ninety-eight pounds four years ago, says he has regained only fifteen pounds and attributes his success to "eating Micro meals every day and learning what not to eat." He recalls the day he decided to diet, "I was looking out my eighth-floor apartment window, pondering my future. It did not look good. I was sixty-five years old and grotesquely overweight—one hundred pounds. Then I was introduced to the program by an Advisor."

John began to notice results almost immediately. "I could not believe my eyes as the fat seemed to disintegrate off my body. I got rid of ninety-eight pounds of ugly fat in less then one year, and I've started dating again. Who said life is over at sixty-five? That's when I started my new life."

Let me show you just how easy it is for John and anyone else who doesn't like cooking to prepare the loser-friendly Micro meals:

**Drinks and soups:** Micro shakes and soups dissolve easily and are excellent hot or cold. Add the mix to water (not the other way round). To mix a smooth, creamy drink or hearty soup, use a blender (if you don't mind the additional washing up). A hand blender is just as effective and easier to clean (put the mixture into the blender before turning on, otherwise you might plaster the ceiling with food). There are plastic shakers on the market which, with a little vigorous shaking, will do the job. (Another word of caution: using hot liquid or carbonated beverages can literally have an explosive effect, so proceed with caution when shaking.)

A wire spring whisk with a bowl or even a clean, screw-top jar (a coffee jar, for instance) can also be used to mix the drinks. To retain most of the nutrients, consume the meal immediately.

**Breakfast cereal:** You can enjoy the traditional European muesli hot or cold, and at any time of the day. Simply put the cereal into a bowl and add water (the milk is already in the mix). The amount of water you add is up to you, although most people prefer to add one to two cups—twice as much as you would use for a drink or soup. Stir, and eat!

**Bars:** Here's a meal everyone can fix. Susan Meyerott, author of the lifestyle enhancement program, *Choices*, came up with this simple two-step procedure: open wrapper; insert bar in mouth.

**Entrees:** Instructions will vary slightly from meal to meal (and are contained on each individual packet) but all are ready in ten minutes or less. Essentially all that you have to do is take boiling water, pour over the meal, and stir. Leave for a couple of minutes so that the ingredients can rehydrate, stir again, possibly leave a little longer, and then eat.

## *THE FOOD DIARY*

Let's acknowledge right away that record-keeping can be a boring task. But it's also really important. Meticulously keeping a daily record of what you eat and drink will help you to become more aware of your personal eating habits. Fill in the diary no matter which of the diet plans you opt to follow.

Note each time you have a Micro meal and write down any other food and drink which you may consume. Also, note down the time and "reason": Did you have ice cream at three P.M. because you were really hungry? Did you eat it without thinking because someone offered it to you? Or were you bored, angry, upset, or anxious? Note, too, the times you're most hungry so you can adjust meal times accordingly.

Very often we are unaware of why we overeat. Keeping a daily record will reveal your personal eating pattern. Once you have identified that pattern and the reason behind it, you are already on the road to healthier eating.

Marion Lampman meticulously kept a food diary during the five-and-a-half months it took her to lose fifty-five pounds, a period which included a six-week Christmas celebration and a New Year's vacation. Says Marion, who has maintained her goal weight for two years, "It became a real fun project for me. I think it is incredibly important to be aware of what we are eating and the effect it has on our bodies. I have learned so much about me and my body during this dieting experience. I think it's necessary to keep a daily chart of one's measurements—bust, waist, and hips as well as weight—because if someone is faithfully following The Micro Diet they may well be losing inches, even if they are not losing pounds."

From day one of her diet, Marion chose to add a banana to her breakfast shake, and turned to an apple if she felt the need to nibble during the evening. For most of the weight-loss regimen she elected to follow the Two Plus One plan, and she also discovered the joys of exercise. "One thing I do religiously is walk two miles a day. I treat it like brushing my teeth. If I don't exercise, I feel like I'm missing something. I feel like I forgot to brush my teeth. I actually worked up to walking three or four miles a day, and then realized my body didn't need to be pushed so much. I learned that if you try to do too much, you get burned out. That's why so many people quit an exercise program. I feel you just need to do enough to be effective for you."

Sixty-three-year-old Marion, a real estate broker in Anchorage, Alaska, was 185 pounds when she first encountered The Micro Diet, and she describes herself as a stress eater. "I thought that at my age the best I could do was take off some of the bulk. I never dreamed I could find the figure of a twenty-year-old down underneath it all and have a twenty-six-inch waist again. I was amazed at how evenly the weight came off. The dieting did not cause any sagging skin and my face does not look haggard."

From an "ill-fitting size sixteen, pushing eighteen," Marion slimmed down to a size eight. "I am more attractive. I am healthier. I feel better and I have much more energy. My kids are proud of me and I can wear prettier clothes. I even went and purchased a new bathing suit. I have not been ashamed to go lie in the sun (yes, we have sun in Alaska), and have a wonderful tan for the first time in years. I know the word is to stay out of the sun but I could not resist. With my new shape it seemed I should have that 'finishing touch'."

Muff Juber is another successful dieter who found that keeping a diary was an extremely valuable tool. "I came to realize that getting overtired triggered uncontrolled binging. So when I feel tired or grumpy I force myself to rest, drink extra water, or go for a walk, depending upon the circumstances. These all seemed to relieve the desire to browse around in the kitchen."

Write down everything that you eat...that lump of cheese, that handful of peanuts. Calories lurk everywhere. Are you chewing gum instead of "eating"? Some chewing gum holds ten calories per stick. Just five sticks a day, seven days a week equals 350 calories. It all adds up.

## *EATING THE BASIC FOUR*

(Food Diary)

| Food Eaten | Amount | Milk | Meat | Fruits & Veg | Grains | Others |
|---|---|---|---|---|---|---|
| | | | | | | |
| Total number of servings from each group | | | | | | |
| Your Goal is (For nonpregnant or nonlactating women) | | 2 | 2 | 4 | 4 | |

Serving size:

**Milk:** 1 Cup milk, yogurt, or equivalent (1½ ounce cheese, 2 Cups cottage cheese).

**Meat:** 2 ounces lean meat, fish, poultry, or cheese, 2 eggs, ½ Cup cottage cheese, 1 Cup dried beans or peas.

**Fruit–Vegetable:** ½ Cup cooked or juice; 1 Cup raw, portion commonly used—medium-sized fruit.

**Grains:** 1 Slice bread, 1 Cup uncooked cereal, ½ Cup cooked cereal, ½ Cup cooked pasta.

## EATING DIARY

| Food Eaten | | Alone? | Eating Partners? | Time | Place of Eating | COMMENTS (*mood, what thinking, feeling, experiencing, etc., i.e., "feel antsy"*) | Other Activities While Eating |
|---|---|---|---|---|---|---|---|
| Type | Quantity | | | | | | |
| | | | | | | | |

## ■ A CASE STUDY
## DR. DENIS WAITLEY: A HIGH-TECH MEAL

For over twenty-seven years, renowned self-esteem speaker, Dr. Denis Waitley, has taught behavior modification. He's trained and counseled Olympic athletes, astronauts, top executives, and prisoners of war to overcome fears and negative conditioning, and to get the most they can out of life.

For years, he says, he has faced his own personal struggle as a different kind of P.O.W. "The initials P.O.W. to me have signified both Putting On Weight and Prisoner of Weight," he says. "During the past few years, I've gone from the body of a football half-back to that of a third-string lineman of a last-place team. I've hovered around the 200-pound mark and reached the point where I started wearing my sports shirt outside of my trousers rather than tucked in." The years of travelling on the international lecture circuit, eating on airplanes, sitting at the head table at banquets, and snacking on the run had taken their toll.

"I decided to take action and start being a real role model and walking testimony of my own teaching of 'The Psychology of Winning,' and I had to choose a nutrition and total fitness program that really works and that people can trust." Dr. Waitley chose The Micro Diet and, using Micro meals to replace some of his "on the run" eating, managed to lose ten pounds in two months. "With my busy schedule it's really amazing how well I've done," he says. "I believe in The Micro Diet because it's the only program I've found that effectively combines the three necessary factors that a successful diet should have. First, it has nutritious, great-tasting meals to help you take the weight off. Secondly, it offers a fun-to-do exercise program. And thirdly, the behavior modification programs offered through the Advisor support network combine motivation and self-image enhancement to give you healthy choices to make instead of chances to take.

"Currently, I am on the Two Plus One plan. I have The Micro Diet for breakfast and lunch, and an early dinner with my wife, family, or friends. This approach allows me to take the weight off slowly while enjoying social functions. I also like to alternate Micro meals for breakfast. One morning I'll have a bowl of Micro muesli by simply adding water. The next morning I'll select a chocolate shake. For lunch, I'll alternate between a bowl of Micro soup and a micro bar. I love all the Micro foods, including the international cuisine."

Adds Dr. Waitley, "In time, the good habits you'll gain from the Micro Diet program will become so enjoyable and second nature, like brushing your teeth or driving your car, that the old bad habits will be overridden and discarded. I tell Micro Dieters, 'Think of your body as a Ferrari. It's a high-powered, high-tech, superbly styled, sleek, finely engineered transportation vehicle. When you put Micro meals into your fuel tank, think of each meal as a high-performance pit stop. Each Micro meal gives you a high-tech, complete performance meal without having to worry or count calories. Your health is the most precious gift of all. It is the one commodity that we don't recognize and appreciate, until it leaves us. Your health, your wellness, and your success are now in your reach and, more, in your control. Stick with The Micro Diet. You deserve to join us in the winner's circle.'"

# 7

# THE 800–1,000 CALORIE PLAN

FOR CONVENIENT, FAST WEIGHT LOSS many dieters choose to follow the 800–1,000 calorie plan eating only Micro meals for breakfast, lunch, dinner, and when snacking. The result is a satisfying weight loss of well over ten pounds a month. Micro Dieters commonly refer to this as going "sole source" because, in this regimen, Micro meals are often the dieter's *sole* source of nutrition. As I explained earlier, this plan is really "loser-friendly" because it takes all of the guesswork out of dieting. You don't have to count calories, weigh foods, or worry about portion control: it's all done for you. It provides good-tasting nutrition with less fat and calories than you would obtain in other foods. In fact, it would be extremely difficult to obtain such nourishment selecting even the healthiest foods off a supermarket shelf.

Micro meals contain from 175–295 calories. Dieters, therefore, can either enjoy these meals alone or select three meals and add healthy snacks, such as fruit and vegetables, to ensure they consume 800 calories and, if they wish, to raise their fiber intake.

Women can obtain their protein RDA of forty-four grams per day by picking *any* three Micro meals. Men need to pick any *four* Micro meals or check the protein content of each meal to choose combinations which add up to their RDA of fifty-six grams (or add other foods containing protein).

The following comparisons of calorie, protein, fat, and sodium content vividly illustrate the benefits of selecting Micro meals over "traditional" meals. At the end of this section you'll find a three-week 800–1,000 calorie "sole source" plan. You can follow these examples exactly as outlined, or you can "mix and match" Micro meals according to your personal preference.

## BREAKFAST

How do typical breakfast meals compare with Micro meals? Just look at the nutritional information in these typical breakfasts and check against the content of the Micro meals. (In these examples you don't add anything to the Micro meals except water.)

### You've Got to Make Sure You Get Enough Protein for Breakfast

**Eggs, Toast, and Juice**

2 slices toast
2 pats butter
1 cup orange juice
1 fried egg

**Micro Vanilla Drink**

1 packet Micro Vanilla Drink, prepared with 1–2 cups water

or

**Micro Hot Chocolate**

1 packet Micro Chocolate Drink, prepared with 1–2 cups hot water

or

**Micro Strawberry Shake**

1 packet Micro Strawberry Drink prepared with 1–2 cups ice water

*Nutritional Information for Typical and Micro Meal Breakfast*

PER TYPICAL BREAKFAST
Calories: 410
Protein: 12 grams
Fat: 17 grams (38%)
Sodium: 1085 mg

PER MICRO DRINK BREAKFAST
Calories: 210
Protein: 22 grams
Fat: 2 grams (9%)
Sodium: 500 mg
Provides 35% RDA of vitamins, minerals, and trace elements.

***The Comparison***

You may find it hard to believe but you enjoy almost twice as much high-quality protein from a Micro drink than from an egg breakfast. That's because Micro drinks are made out of nonfat milk, egg whites, and other good foodstuff. This provides you with high-quality protein in half the calories and less than 10% fat. All Micro drinks can be served hot, cold, or chilled.

## Nothing Is Healthier than Oatmeal...Or Is It?

**Oatmeal, Fruit, and Juice**

1 cup cooked oatmeal
½ cup 2% milk
1 banana, sliced
½ cup orange juice

**Micro Muesli Cereal***

1 packet muesli cereal, prepared with 1–2 cups water

*The Micro muesli mix already contains nonfat milk, raisins, nuts, and oats.

*Nutritional Information for Typical and Micro Meal Breakfast*

PER OATMEAL BREAKFAST
Calories: 366
Protein: 12 grams
Fat: 6 grams (13%)
Fiber: 1 gram
Sodium: 384 mg

PER MICRO MUESLI BREAKFAST
Calories: 260
Protein: 17 grams
Fat: 4 grams (14%)
Fiber: 8 grams
Sodium: 500 mg
Provides 35% RDA of vitamins, minerals, and trace elements.

***The Comparison***
What could be healthier than oatmeal, fruit, and juice for breakfast? The answer is a bowl of Micro muesli! As you can see, Micro muesli packs much more protein, fiber, and nutrients into fewer calories and fat. Because you get more nutrition in fewer calories, you can use The Micro Diet as your sole source of nutrition, eat fewer than 1,000 calories a day, lose weight quickly, and improve your health.

## I Need Something Quick for Breakfast—Just Some Toast and Juice

**Toast and Juice**

2 slices toast
2 pats butter
1 large glass orange juice

**Micro Muesli bar**

1 Micro Bar

*Nutritional Information for Typical and Micro Meal Breakfast*

PER TOAST & JUICE BREAKFAST
Calories: 319
Protein: 6 grams
Fat: 10 grams (29%)
Fiber: less than 1 gram
Sodium: 342 mg

PER MICRO MUESLI BREAKFAST BAR
Calories: 280
Protein: 15 grams
Fat: 4 grams (13%)
Fiber: 6 grams
Sodium: 200 mg
Provides 35% RDA of vitamins, minerals, and trace elements

***The Comparison***

Both breakfasts provide you with something to crunch, reasonable calories, and less than 30% fat for the meal. But the muesli bar takes no time to prepare, and provides you with twice as much high-quality protein, half the fat, six times the fiber, and 35% of the recommended dietary allowances (RDA) for all known vitamins, minerals, and trace elements. Each Micro bar is a complete meal in itself. There's nothing to fix. You simply open the wrapper and eat, making it the perfect "on the go" meal.

# LUNCH

## LUNCH ON THE RUN

**Peanut Butter & Jelly Sandwich**

2 slices bread
2 T peanut butter
1 T jelly

**Micro Peanut Bar**

1 Micro bar

*Nutritional Information for "Lunch on the Run"*

PER SANDWICH
Calories: 368
Fat: 18 grams (43%)
Fiber: 1.6 grams
Sodium: 388 mg

PER MICRO PEANUT BAR
Calories: 260
Fat: 6 grams (21%)
Fiber: 8 grams
Sodium: 500 mg
Provides 35% RDA of vitamins, minerals, and trace elements.

***The Comparison***
We tend to think of a peanut butter and jelly sandwich as a quick-fix meal. But what could be faster than a Micro bar? When you're in a hurry, you grab a Micro bar, put it in your briefcase, pocket or purse, and go. When it's time to eat, all you have to do is "open wrapper and insert bar in mouth"! But the Micro bars are more than convenient, they're healthier, too. That peanut butter sandwich has less fiber, and more fat and calories than the Micro Peanut Bar (or any of the other Micro bars).

Yes, you could use less peanut butter in your sandwich. But the issue isn't what you could do, but what you normally do. When you take a long, hard look at what you actually do eat on an everyday basis and compare with the Micro meals, it's easy to see why The Micro Diet enhances your health as you lose weight. On The Micro Diet you lower the fat and calories, while raising the nutritional quality of your meals.

## BAG LUNCHES (Home Prepared)

**Tuna Sandwich "Bag" Lunch**

Tuna sandwich made with tuna (canned in water), light mayonnaise, pickle relish
1 glass 2% milk
banana

**Micro Chocolate Bar**

1 Micro bar

*Nutritional Information for Bag Lunch*

PER TUNA "BAG" LUNCH
- Calories: 605
- Protein: 37 grams
- Fat: 22 grams (31%)
- Fiber: 1.5 grams
- Sodium: 898 mg

PER MICRO CHOCOLATE BAR
- Calories: 280
- Protein: 16 grams
- Fat: 9 grams (27%)
- Fiber: 5 grams
- Sodium: 100 mg

Provides 35% RDA of vitamins, minerals, and trace elements.

### *The Comparison*

Having a tuna sandwich, made with light mayonnaise and water-packed tuna, is a good homemade choice for lunch. But, this "healthy" lunch contains twice the calories and fat as the Micro Chocolate Bar, and only one-third of the fiber. The tuna lunch does have twice as much protein as the Micro Chocolate Bar, but be careful. While you need to have enough high-quality protein, too much isn't good. Men need at least fifty-six grams of protein a day; women forty-four grams. The Micro meals provide you with just enough. Each meal has one-quarter to one-third of the recommended amount for the day. To lose weight on 1,000 calories a day, you should keep your fat intake to thirty-three grams or less. If you eat this tuna sandwich lunch while attempting to lose weight, you consume two-thirds of your calories and fat for the day in one meal. All Micro meals provide no more than ten grams of fat, and no more than 300 calories per meal.

**Ham Sandwich "Bag" Lunch**

Ham sandwich, made with luncheon meat, light mayonnaise, mustard
glass 2% milk
apple
2 chocolate chip cookies

**Micro Chicken Tetrazzini**

1 packet, Micro Chicken Tetrazzini prepared with ¾–1 cup hot water

*Nutritional Information for "Bag" Lunch*

PER HAM SANDWICH "BAG" LUNCH
Calories: 587
Protein: 24 grams
Fat: 21 grams (33%)
Fiber: 1.5 grams
Sodium: 1291 mg

PER MICRO CHICKEN TETRAZZINI
Calories: 260
Protein: 21 grams
Fat: 1 gram (3%)
Fiber: less than 1 gram
Sodium: 840 mg
Provides 35% RDA of vitamins, minerals, and trace elements

***The Comparison***
The ham sandwich is still a favorite of many people. With The Micro Diet you can enjoy a ham sandwich some of the time. We just don't recommend it all of the time. Notice you'd have to eat about nineteen servings of Micro Chicken Tetrazzini before you consumed as much fat as there is in the ham sandwich lunch. There's only two thin slices of luncheon ham in this meal, but there's also fat lurking in the light mayonnaise, low-fat milk, and cookies. You could actually eat two servings of the chicken tetrazzini for the same number of calories you get in the entire bag lunch. That's why many people can add other foods to the Micro meals and still lose weight.

**Campbell's Tomato Soup**

1 can, prepared with milk

**Micro Diet's Creamy Tomato Soup**

1 packet, prepared with 1–2 cups water

*Nutritional Information for Tomato Soup Lunch*

PER CAMPBELL'S TOMATO SOUP
Calories: 320
Protein: 12 grams
Fat: 12 grams (32%)
Fiber: 1 gram
Sodium: 1864 mg

PER MICRO TOMATO SOUP
Calories: 244
Protein: 20 grams
Fat: 4 grams (15%)
Fiber: 1 gram
Sodium: 700 mg
Provides 35% RDA of vitamins, minerals, and trace elements.

***The Comparison***
Campbell's Tomato Soup is one of the best-selling soups in America. It's tasty and it's a good source of protein when prepared with milk, as well as being an excellent source of vitamin A and vitamin C. But it still can't measure up to The Micro Diet Creamy Tomato Soup, which provides 35% of the RDA for all known vitamins, minerals, and trace elements in addition to providing more high-quality protein in fewer

calories. The Micro Diet creamy tomato soup mix contains nonfat milk, and provides excellent taste and nutrition.

**Lipton Green Pea Cup-A-Soup**

1 Package

**Micro Diet Hearty Pea Soup**

1 packet, prepared with 1–2 cups water

*Nutritional Information for Pea Soup "Lunch"*

PER LIPTON GREEN PEA CUP
Calories: 80
Protein: 2 grams
Fat: 4 grams (45%)
Fiber: less than 1 gram
Sodium: 820 mg

PER MICRO DIET PEA SOUP
Calories: 233
Protein: 16 grams
Fat: 5 grams (19%)
Fiber: less than 1 gram
Sodium: 700 mg
Provides 35% RDA of vitamins, minerals, and trace elements

***The Comparison***

The Lipton Green Pea Soup is definitely not designed to be a meal. The protein content is insignificant, as is the amount of vitamins, minerals, and trace elements. It'll warm your stomach and not do much else. Although the Micro pea soup is 233 calories and Lipton's is only 80 calories, 45% of the calories in Lipton's pea soup derive from fat, while only 19% of the Micro pea soup come from fat. And the Micro pea soup, like all Micro meals, provides 35% of your daily requirements and is a complete, filling meal in itself.

## SNACKS

**Roasted Peanuts**

½ cup peanuts

**Peanut Butter Cups (Candy)**

4 peanut butter cups

**Micro Crunchy Peanut Bar**

1 Micro bar

*Nutritional Information for "Snack on the Run"*

PER ½ CUP PEANUTS
Calories: 420
Fat: 36 grams (71%)
Fiber: 1.7 grams
Sodium: 11 mg

PER CRUNCHY PEANUT BAR
Calories: 290
Fat: 10 grams (29%)
Fiber: 4 grams
Sodium: 200 mg
Provides 35% RDA of vitamins, minerals, and trace elements.

PER 4 PEANUT BUTTER CUPS
Calories: 368
Fat: 21 grams (52%)
Fiber: less than 1 gram
Sodium: 218 mg

***The Comparisons***
The Micro Crunchy Peanut Bar is highly popular. Like all other Micro meals, it is designed to be a complete meal, but for those people who aren't reducing their caloric intake to the minimum level (or for anyone interested in healthier eating) it makes a great snack. It tastes like a candy bar, yet it delivers a tremendous nutritional package. Whether you grab for a "healthy" snack of peanuts, with a whopping 71% of the calories coming from fat, or you turn to a "junk" snack of Reese's Peanut Butter Cups, with 52% of the calories coming from fat, you're eating a lot more fat and calories than you would in the Micro bar. All Micro meals contain 30% or less fat.

## QUICK-FIX DINNERS

**Canned Chili Con Carne/Beans**

Open can of Chili, heat, serve.

**Micro Chili**

Heat 1 cup water, add to Micro Chili, and stir. Let stand in covered bowl for 10 minutes.

*Nutritional Information Per Serving*

PER CANNED CHILI
Portion: 1 cup
Calories: 340
Fat: 16 grams (42%)
Fiber: 1.5 grams
Sodium: 1354 mg

PER MICRO CHILI
Portion: 1 packet
Calories: 210
Fat: .5 grams (2%)
Fiber: 4 grams
Sodium: 600 mg
Provides 35% RDA of vitamins, minerals, and trace elements

***The Comparison***
To lose weight and improve your health the most important change you can make in your diet is to lower the fat, especially animal fat. All Micro meals are combination foods made out of foods such as nonfat milk, soybeans, oats, egg whites, wheat, currants, and raisins. They are

primarily based in plant and low- or non-fat animal products. What you can see in the comparison above is that the Micro Chili is significantly lower in fat, calories, and sodium, and higher in fiber than the canned chili. What you can't see is the fact that the canned chili con carne contains beef and is high in saturated fat, while the plant-based Micro chili is low in saturated fat. Saturated fat, found primarily in animal fat, is the biggest culprit for raising blood cholesterol. All Micro meals are very low in saturated fat and cholesterol. It's easy to get lazy at the end of the day and just grab something that tastes good—like a can of chili—that doesn't provide complete nutrition. Micro meals make it easy to grab good taste and good nutrition every time.

**Grilled Cheese Sandwich Dinner**

2 pieces whole-wheat bread
3 ounces Cheddar cheese
1 tablespoon butter
1 glass 2% milk
1 apple

**Micro Spanish Rice Dinner**

1 packet, prepared with ¾–1¼ cup hot water
Let stand 10 minutes in covered bowl.

*Nutritional Information for Quick-Fix Dinner*

PER GRILLED CHEESE DINNER
Calories: 781
Protein: 35 grams
Fat: 47 grams (53%)
Fiber: 2 grams
Sodium: 1122 mg

PER MICRO SPANISH RICE DINNER
Calories: 260
Protein: 17 grams
Fat: 2 grams (7%)
Fiber: 2 grams
Sodium: 750 mg
Provides 35% RDA of vitamins, minerals, and trace elements

### *The Comparison*

To lose weight on a 1,000-calorie-a-day diet, you should consume no more than thirty-three grams of fat (30% of total calories for the day). The grilled cheese dinner contains forty-seven grams of fat, or 53% of the dinner calories! This is way over the recommended limit for the entire day! The Micro Spanish Rice, with just two grams of fat, leaves you thirty-one grams of fat for your breakfast and lunch meals, making it easier to keep your fat intake to 30% or less of your total calories for the day. While it's important to have enough high-quality protein in your diet, too much isn't good. Micro meals, including the Spanish rice, provide one-quarter to one-third of the recommended dietary allowances (RDA) for protein in each meal. At thirty-five grams of protein, the grilled cheese dinner is excessive.

**Quesadilla Dinner**

2 flour tortillas
⅓ cup shredded Cheddar cheese
½ cup refried beans
1 glass 2% milk

**Micro Creamy Chicken Soup**

1 packet prepared with 1–2 cups hot water

*Nutritional Information for Quick-Fix Dinners*

PER QUESADILLA DINNER
Calories: 596
Protein: 30 grams
Fat: 22 grams (33%)
Fiber: 4 grams
Sodium: 889 mg

PER MICRO CREAMY CHICKEN SOUP
Calories: 175
Protein: 19 grams
Fat: 4 grams (20%)
Fiber: less than 1 gram
Sodium: 625 mg
Provides 35% RDA of vitamins, minerals, and trace elements

***The Comparison***

The quesadilla dinner isn't too bad, as dinner meals go. But it has more protein and fat than necessary, and a lot less nutrition than the Micro chicken soup. And look what happens if you take seconds: A double serving of the quesadilla dinner costs you 1,192 calories and forty-four grams of fat, while a double serving of the Micro chicken soup dinner costs you 350 calories and eight grams of fat. Or you could have Micro Spanish rice and Micro Creamy chicken soup for dinner for only 435 calories and six grams of fat (21%)—and still eat three times less fat than you'd consume in the single-portion quesadilla dinner.

## *SUMMARY*

Because all Micro meals are combination foods that provide you with a balance of nutrients, you can be assured of proper nutrition when you select any one of them. You don't have to eat a particular meal at any particular time. You can have chili for breakfast if you want, or muesli cereal for dinner. It's up to you. Most people find that they vastly prefer certain meals and, in spite of the variety available, tend to eat those personal favorites more frequently. Doesn't that hold true for nondieters as well? It's your choice. As a general rule, however, it's a good idea to eat a variety of foods.

## *DAILY MENU*

### *A Comparison of a Typical Meal Plan and a Micro Diet 800–1,000 Calorie "Sole Source" Plan*

| Typical | Micro |
|---|---|
| ***BREAKFAST*** | |
| Fried Egg<br>Toast<br>Orange Juice | Micro Vanilla Drink |
| ***LUNCH*** | |
| Peanut Butter & Jelly Sandwich | Micro Peanut Bar |
| ***SNACK*** | |
| Roasted Peanuts | Micro Crunchy Peanut Bar |
| ***DINNER*** | |
| Grilled Cheese Sandwich<br>Glass Milk<br>Apple | Micro Spanish Rice |

| DAILY TOTAL TYPICAL MEALS | DAILY TOTAL MICRO MEALS |
|---|---|
| Calories: 1801 | Calories: 1020 |
| Protein: 69 grams | Protein 69 grams |
| Fat: 104 grams (50%) | Fat: 20 grams (17%) |
| Fiber: 5.6 grams | Fiber: 14 grams |
| Sodium: 2606 mg | Sodium: 1950 mg |

SUMMARY:

1. Why can some people lose weight on The Micro Diet when they have difficulty losing on most 1,000–1,200 calorie-a-day diets? Because the Micro meals are so low in fat. If you want to lose weight faster, drop the fat in your diet, but keep the carbohydrates up. The typical daily diet above gets 50% of its calories from fat, while The Micro Diet plan above only gets 17% of its calories from fat.
2. The average American consumes 4,000–6,000 mg of sodium a day. Health professionals recommend we keep our sodium intake under 3,300 mg per day. The daily total for The Micro Diet plan above is well within that limit. Typical combinations of three to four Micro meals will provide you with 1,500–2,700 mg—well within the recommended range.

## *DAILY TOTALS*

### *A Comparison of a Typical Daily Diet with a Micro Diet Menu*

| | |
|---|---|
| ***BREAKFAST*** | |
| Oatmeal<br>Milk<br>Banana<br>Orange Juice | Micro Muesli |
| ***LUNCH*** | |
| Tuna Fish Sandwich<br>Milk<br>Banana | Micro Chocolate Bar |
| ***SNACK*** | |
| Reese's Peanut Butter Cups | Micro Crunchy Peanut Bar |
| ***DINNER*** | |
| Quesadilla<br>Refried Beans<br>Soup<br>Milk | Micro Creamy Chicken Soup |
| DAILY TOTAL<br>Calories: 1773<br>Protein: 83 grams<br>Fat: 64 grams (32%)<br>Fiber: 6 grams<br>Sodium: 1751 mg | DAILY TOTAL<br>Calories: 1005<br>Protein: 67 grams<br>Fat: 27 grams (24%)<br>Fiber: 17 grams<br>Sodium: 1825 mg |

SUMMARY

Like most diets, the typical day starts out good enough, but slowly adds more fat. For a maintenance diet, the typical day isn't bad, but it still gets 32% of the calories from fat. The Micro Diet menu keeps the total calories well within the "losing" range of 1,000 calories, and only gets 24% of the calories from fat. This makes it easier to lose weight.

## COMPARISON OF TYPICAL DIET DAY WITH MICRO DIET DAY

| | |
|---|---|
| ***BREAKFAST*** | |
| Toast<br>Orange Juice | Micro Muesli Bar |
| ***LUNCH*** | |
| Ham Sandwich<br>Milk<br>Apple<br>Cookies | Micro Chicken Tetrazzini |
| ***DINNER*** | |
| Chili Con Carne | Micro Chili |

DAILY TOTAL (TYPICAL DAY)
Calories: 1291
Protein: 49 grams
Fat: 52 grams (36%)
Sodium: 3052 mg

DAILY TOTAL FOR MICRO DIET MENU
Calories: 750
Protein: 51 grams
Fat: 5.5 grams (6%)
Sodium: 1640 mg

SUMMARY

The total calories for the typical day isn't bad, but you have to wonder whether you got adequate nutrition for the day. And, while the total fat intake for the day isn't extremely high, it's about the American average of 37% fat—well above the recommended level of 30% or less. With the Micro Diet plan, you know that with each meal you received 35% of the recommended dietary allowance for all known nutrients, and a proper balance of protein, carbohydrate, and fat. At 750 calories for the day, and only 6% of those calories coming from fat, you can easily afford to add raw vegetables or fruit to your diet and still lose weight. (We do recommend you consume at least 800 calories a day.)

## *SAMPLE 800–1,000 CALORIE "SOLE SOURCE" MENU*

## *WEEK 1*

| MON | TUES | WED | THUR | FRI | SAT | SUN |
|---|---|---|---|---|---|---|
| | | | ***BREAKFAST*** | | | |
| Peanut Bar | Muesli Bar | Chocolate Drink | Yogurt-Orange Bar | Muesli Cereal | Chocolate Bar | Vanilla Drink |
| | | | ***LUNCH*** | | | |
| Tomato Soup | Pea Soup | Crunchy Peanut Bar | Strawberry Drink | Peanut Bar | Chicken Tetrazzini | Crunchy Peanut Bar |
| | | | ***DINNER*** | | | |
| Spanish Rice | Chili | Chicken Soup | Pea Soup | Tomato Soup | Spanish Rice | Chicken Tetrazzini |
| | | | ***SNACK*** | | | |
| ½ Crunchy Peanut Bar | Chocolate Drink | Strawberry Drink | ½ Crunchy Peanut Bar | Vanilla Drink | Chicken Soup | Chocolate Drink |

## *DAILY TOTALS*

| MON | TUES | WED | THUR | FRI | SAT | SUN |
|---|---|---|---|---|---|---|
| | | | ***CALORIES*** | | | |
| 909 cal | 933 cal | 862 cal | 878 cal | 974 cal | 952 cal | 970 cal |
| | | | ***PROTEIN (GRAMS)*** | | | |
| 59 gms | 68 gms | 84 gms | 60 gms | 74 gms | 79 gms | 80 gms |
| | | | ***FAT (GRAMS)*** | | | |
| 17 gms | 12 gms | 15 gms | 21 gms | 16 gms | 13 gms | 15 gms |
| | | | ***% FAT*** | | | |
| 17% | 11% | 16% | 21% | 15% | 12% | 14% |
| | | | ***FIBER (GRAMS)*** | | | |
| 13 gms | 11 gms | 4 gms | 7 gms | 17 gms | 7 gms | 4 gms |
| | | | ***SODIUM (MILLIGRAMS)*** | | | |
| 2050 mg | 2000 mg | 1975 mg | 1400 mg | 2200 mg | 2465 mg | 2040 mg |

## *SAMPLE 800–1,000 CALORIE "SOLE SOURCE" MENU*

## *WEEK 2*

| MON | TUES | WED | THUR | FRI | SAT | SUN |
|---|---|---|---|---|---|---|
| | | | ***BREAKFAST*** | | | |
| Hot Chocolate Drink | Hot Muesli Cereal | Hot Strawberry Drink | Vanilla Drink with ½ Peanut Bar | Yogurt-Orange Bar | Tomato Soup | Hot Muesli Cereal |
| | | | ***LUNCH*** | | | |
| Crunchy Peanut Bar | Peanut Bar | Spanish Rice | Chicken Tetrazzini | Chocolate Drink | Muesli Bar | Strawberry Drink |
| | | | ***DINNER*** | | | |
| Pea Soup | Chicken Soup | Crunchy Peanut Bar | Strawberry Drink | Spanish Rice | Pea Soup | Chicken Tetrazzini |
| | | | ***SNACK*** | | | |
| ½ Chocolate Bar | ½ Chocolate Drink | Chicken Soup | ½ Crunchy Peanut Bar | Pea Soup | ½ Crunchy Peanut Bar | ½ Crunchy Peanut Bar |

## *DAILY TOTALS*

| MON | TUES | WED | THUR | FRI | SAT | SUN |
|---|---|---|---|---|---|---|
| | | | ***CALORIES*** | | | |
| 873 cal | 812 cal | 912 cal | 970 cal | 993 cal | 902 cal | 875 cal |
| | | | ***PROTEIN (GRAMS)*** | | | |
| 61 gms | 65 gms | 74 gms | 80 gms | 70 gms | 59 gms | 68 gms |
| | | | ***FAT (GRAMS)*** | | | |
| 22 gms | 16 gms | 15 gms | 15 gms | 18 gms | 18 gms | 12 gms |
| | | | ***% FAT*** | | | |
| 21% | 17% | 15% | 14% | 16% | 18% | 12% |
| | | | ***FIBER (GRAMS)*** | | | |
| 7 gms | 19 gms | 6 gms | 4 gms | 7 gms | 10 gms | 10 gms |
| | | | ***SODIUM (MILLIGRAMS)*** | | | |
| 1450 mg | 1825 mg | 2225 mg | 2040 mg | 2050 mg | 1700 mg | 1940 mg |

## *SAMPLE 800–1,000 CALORIE "SOLE SOURCE" MENU*

## *WEEK 3*

| MON | TUES | WED | THUR | FRI | SAT | SUN |
|---|---|---|---|---|---|---|
| | | | ***BREAKFAST*** | | | |
| Pea Soup | Chicken Soup | Muesli Bar | Tomato Soup | Chocolate Bar | Vanilla Drink | Peanut Bar |
| | | | ***LUNCH*** | | | |
| Chili | Crunchy Peanut Bar | Chocolate Drink | Chicken Tetrazzini | Pea Soup | Crunchy Peanut Bar | Strawberry Drink |
| | | | ***DINNER*** | | | |
| Spanish Rice | Chicken Tetrazzini | Pea Soup | Chili | Spanish Rice | Chicken Soup | Chili |
| | | | ***SNACK*** | | | |
| ½ Crunchy Peanut Bar | ½ Yogurt-Orange Bar | ½ Crunchy Peanut Bar | Chicken Soup | ½ Yogurt-Orange Bar | ½ Chocolate Bar | ½ Chocolate Bar |

## *DAILY TOTALS*

| MON | TUES | WED | THUR | FRI | SAT | SUN |
|---|---|---|---|---|---|---|
| | | | ***CALORIES*** | | | |
| 848 cal | 847 cal | 868 cal | 866 cal | 918 cal | 800 cal | 820 cal |
| | | | ***PROTEIN (GRAMS)*** | | | |
| 56 gms | 68 gms | 61 gms | 81 gms | 57 gms | 70 gms | 60 gms |
| | | | ***FAT (GRAMS)*** | | | |
| 13 gms | 17 gms | 16 gms | 7 gms | 21 gms | 18 gms | 13 gms |
| | | | ***% FAT*** | | | |
| 13% | 18% | 16% | 7% | 20% | 20% | 14% |
| | | | ***FIBER (GRAMS)*** | | | |
| 9 gms | 6 gms | 9 gms | 5 gms | 10 gms | 7 gms | 15 gms |
| | | | ***SODIUM (MILLIGRAMS)*** | | | |
| 2150 mg | 1915 mg | 1500 mg | 2915 mg | 1600 mg | 1525 mg | 1650 mg |

## *VARIETY IS THE SPICE OF LIFE*

Micro meals were designed to be enjoyed straight out of the packet by simply mixing them with water and nothing else. There are plenty of Micro meals suitable for every eating occasion—breakfast, lunch, dinner, supper, and snacks. But variety is the spice of life, and there are many ways to get even more variety out of the Micro Diet range of meals while adding very few calories, or none at all.

How? Quite simply by utilizing a variety of spices, flavorings, and low-calorie sodas to produce different meals to suit your own palate. If you don't mind a few extra calories and want to further change the taste and texture of your meals, you can use orange juice, cocoa, yogurt, or fruit. In fact, anything you want. After all, no matter how much you might like the chocolate drink, for example, you won't want to drink it "straight" three times a day, seven days a week!

Don't make a shake and quickly chug it down, or eat your chili standing at the kitchen sink. Experiment making a Micro meal a fine dining experience. The way in which you present a meal makes all the difference in the world. We do "eat with our eyes." So serve your shake in a large, attractively shaped glass. Mix with chilled water or crushed ice to make a cool drink or thick shake. Add a strawberry to the strawberry drink, sprinkle some cinnamon on the chocolate. Sip your shake through a straw. Be inventive. Have fun. Serve chicken soup, for example, in a soup bowl, garnished with paprika, parsley, poultry seasoning, marjoram, onion, garlic, sage, thyme, or jalapeno peppers, and sit down at the dinner table with the rest of the family. To get you started, here is a selection of appetizing suggestions for creating some "exotic" Micro meals, which will please your taste buds without disrupting your diet.

## *VANILLA DRINK*

### *Cola Shake*

1 serving Micro Vanilla Drink
8 ounces Diet Coke

### *Apricot Delight*

1 serving Micro Vanilla Drink
8 ounces water
¼ teaspoon apricot flavoring
cinnamon

### *Frozen Daiquiri*

1 serving Micro Vanilla Drink
8 ounces water
½ teaspoon rum essence

### *Pineapple Cream*

1 serving Micro Vanilla Drink
8 ounces water
¼ teaspoon pineapple flavoring

### *Orange Fizz*

1 serving Micro Vanilla Drink
4 ounces orange juice
Water to taste

### *Caribbean Cocktail*

1 serving Micro Vanilla Drink
8 ounces water
4 drops pineapple essence
4 drops coconut essence

### *Orange Dream*

1 serving Micro Vanilla Drink
¼ teaspoon orange flavoring
Water to taste

### *Cappuccino*

1 serving Micro Vanilla Drink
1 cup hot water
low-calorie sweetener
1 teaspoon instant decaffeinated coffee
¼ teaspoon rum flavor
⅛ teaspoon cinnamon

### *Pina Colada*

1 serving Micro Vanilla Drink
6 ounces chilled water
1 cup crushed ice
½ packet artificial sweetener
few drops of coconut, pineapple, rum, and orange extracts

## *STRAWBERRY DRINK*

### *Butterberry*

1 serving Micro Strawberry Drink
8 ounces cold water
1 teaspoon butterscotch syrup

### *Caribbean Strawberry*

1 serving Micro Strawberry Drink
8 ounces cold water
¼ teaspoon rum essence

### *Sunny Strawberry Delight*

1 serving Micro Strawberry Drink
8 ounces cold water
1 tablespoon raspberries

### *Strawberry Zest*

1 serving Micro Strawberry Drink
8 ounces cold water
Grated zest of ½ lemon

### *Strawberry Fizz*

1 serving Micro Strawberry Drink
4 ounces cold water
4 ounces Diet 7–Up

### *South Sea Strawberry*

1 serving Micro Strawberry Drink
8 ounces cold water
½ juice from lime

## *CHOCOLATE DRINK*

### *Hot Milk Chocolate*

½ serving Micro Chocolate Drink
½ serving Micro Vanilla Drink
4 ounces cold water
4 ounces hot water

### *Chocolate Orange Supreme*

1 serving Micro Chocolate Drink
8 ounces water
½ teaspoon orange flavoring

### *Chocolate Cola*

1 serving Micro Chocolate Drink
1 cup Diet Coke or diet cola
Water to taste

### *Coconana*

1 serving Micro Chocolate Drink
8 ounces cold water
¼ teaspoon coconut essence

### *Cool Chocolate Mint*

1 serving Micro Chocolate Drink
8 ounces cold water
¼ teaspoon peppermint essence

## *CHICKEN SOUP*

### *Thick Curried Chicken*

1 serving Micro Chicken Soup
8 ounces hot water
¼ teaspoon curry powder
½ teaspoon turmeric

### *Hungarian Chicken*

1 serving Micro Chicken Soup
8 ounces hot water
¼ teaspoon paprika
½ teaspoon garlic puree
½ packet sweetener

### *Chicken Worcester*

1 serving Micro Chicken Soup
8 ounces hot water
½ teaspoon Worcestershire sauce
½ teaspoon onion powder

### *Spring Chicken*

1 serving Micro Chicken Soup
8 ounces hot water
½ teaspoon dried chives
1 stalk chopped parsley

### *Chinese Chicken*

1 serving Micro Chicken Soup
8 ounces hot water
½ teaspoon soy sauce
chopped bean sprouts

### *Middle East Chicken*

1 serving Micro Chicken Soup
8 ounces hot water
½ teaspoon coriander
½ teaspoon garlic puree

### *Chicken and Vegetable*

1 serving Micro Chicken Soup
8 ounces hot water
½ stick celery
1 small grated carrot
¼ teaspoon onion powder

### *Peking Chicken*

1 serving Micro Chicken Soup
8 ounces hot water
¼ teaspoon ginger
½ teaspoon garlic powder
½ teaspoon chives

## ■ A CASE STUDY
## ROBIN LEACH: THE CAVIAR OF DIETS

Robin Leach, star of television's *Lifestyles of the Rich and Famous* had adapted The Micro Diet to suit his own extravagant way of life.

The jet-setting personality who travels 200,000 miles a year and visits the most exquisite restaurants and resorts in the world faces temptation everywhere he goes. Gourmet chefs and maitre d's are always plying him with champagne, caviar, and "the best" that their kitchens have to offer. That often means loads of fattening treats. No wonder that Robin's girth expanded so much that he confesses, "At two hundred and six pounds, I looked about eight months pregnant."

Says Robin, "My experience has been a positive one from the very first moment that I bit into a muesli bar. First of all the variety of food is extraordinary, you don't get bored with this diet. It's almost as if you're not on a diet at all. I lost weight with my doctor's encouragement and I feel I did it sensibly and painlessly, and I had a lot more energy.

"My little daily walk of twenty minutes on the treadmill is now up to one hour, and I could easily do another hour. When I started The Micro Diet, I suddenly found myself getting interested in swimming. I began doing just two laps, I'm up to twelve laps, and the only thing that stops me from doing twenty-four laps is running out of time."

Adds Robin, who has lost twenty-eight pounds with The Micro Diet (twenty-four in the first ten weeks), "It's very tasty. I don't feel like a medieval monk doing penance for lewd thoughts. It was a pain-free way to diet. I would go five days eating nothing but Micro meals and then a few days eating other meals as well, so that it suited my social life. I had a little trick of my own. Every morning with my first cup of tea I would cut my Muesli bar in half and just eat half. I would have the other half as my mid-morning snack.

"I've lost most of the weight from my stomach. Those 'love handles' aren't what they used to be, and it's so heartening to listen to people saying to me, 'Boy, do you look good. You look ten years younger. What's the secret?' I'm now wearing clothes that I haven't been able to wear in five years; they were just hanging in plastic bags at the back of the closet. I do have one wonderful problem. I have to get new belts or have new holes punched in the old ones. I started out with thirty-eight-inch trousers. I'm now down to a thirty-four waist and I've run out of holes in the belt.

"Quite honestly, I have an amazing amount of energy now. I feel better than I have for twenty years. I feel that if I can lose weight with my way of life, anyone can."

# 8

# THE 1,000–1,200 CALORIE PLAN

ARE YOU CONTENT WITH slower weight loss? Would you enjoy an even greater diversity of meals? Do you like experimenting in the kitchen? If you answered "yes" to one of these questions, the 1,000–1,200 calorie plan is for you. You'll discover how just a few extra calories can turn your diet into a delightful gastronomic experience. You'll find out why Micro meals should be an essential ingredient in any self-respecting cook's repertoire. You'll be shown how Micro meals are the perfect foundation for nutritionally well-balanced cooking, not only for dieters but also for everyone interested in healthier eating.

Micro meals are simply combination foods made of wholesome ingredients such as nonfat milk, grains, fruits and vegetables—the kind of food used frequently by executive chefs such as Bill McLeish, of Doraville, Georgia.

Unfortunately for Bill, sugar and fat were even more common ingredients and, after years of testing and tasting his own masterpieces, he became a victim of his own cooking, weighing 279 pounds. But, after losing eighty-four pounds with The Micro Diet, he's converted to the loser-friendly way of life—and has turned his culinary skills toward creating great-tasting, healthy meals.

Forty-year-old Bill, an honors graduate of the Culinary Institute of America, has more than twenty years, experience in the food-service industry including hotels, fine dining restaurants, and private clubs. During his career he has prepared gourmet meals featuring ingredients from all over the world. He has overseen food preparation for groups as large as 10,000 people, and he even cooked for President Gerald Ford.

"There's a slogan in the restaurant business: Never trust a skinny chef. I was very trustworthy," says Bill with a chuckle, since he can now afford to laugh about his former self. But, back in the fall of 1990, he says, "I was a very unhappy, depressed, unmotivated, 'feeling like a failure' person. My zest for life had disappeared. It was getting to be a challenge each day just to get out of bed to face the next hardship.

"My eating habits had grown out of control because eating was something I could get pleasure from, but the sugar overdoses were throwing me into an emotional tailspin. Unpredictable mood swings were affecting my personal relationships. My family never knew what to expect from me."

As an executive chef, Bill says that he always took pride in producing the tastiest, richest meals he could create. "The first step in preparing any meal was to melt a pot of butter on the back burner. I didn't realize the damage I was doing to my family, friends, customers, and myself by cooking with excessive amounts of fats and calories."

Running a catering service out of his home made matters worse for Bill and his family. Because he was "too busy," they ate all of the tasty leftovers—mainly sweets. Bill, wife Susan, and son Doug, all ballooned to their heaviest weights. Then Susan was introduced to The Micro Diet and immediately began to see results. That was all the encouragement Bill needed. Within a week he was following his wife's example. Doug followed soon afterward.

It was November 1990 and the McLeish family set themselves a goal: to lose an entire "person" by Easter. They decided that meant getting rid of at least a hundred pounds. When Easter came, the threesome showed a collective, impressive weight loss of 140 pounds: Bill (sixty), Susan (forty-three), and Doug (thirty-seven).

"It was an opportunity for me to be creative and healthy at the same time," says Bill. "I feel that a big factor in my family's weight loss has been the variety I have been able to bring to the preparation of meals. We have found my recipes to play a very important role in the experience of our dieters.

"My zest for life has returned, my self-confidence is at an all-time high, my love for cooking has returned, and my mood swings have leveled out. For the first time in a long time I feel successful. I want to help dieters learn how to use The Micro Diet to its fullest potential. With a little extra knowledge and effort, these products can become lifelong 'friends.'"

The recipes which Bill created and which helped his family to lose weight are presented here to help you. Many people, of course, prefer to use meals straight out of the packet for convenience and because they taste so good. But if you like to cook (and most people don't hate to cook, they hate to *have to* cook), experiment with Bill's suggestions, and you will discover an amazing variety of culinary opportunities. These "enhancements" to the basic Micro meals all keep to the basic principles of high nutrition, low fat (less than 30% calories from fat).

Bill has covered all of the bases: There are ways to use Micro meals to make cookies, pies, crepes, chowder, soups, and dips. There are hors d'oeuvres, stews, salads, puddings, even a pizza dish. Whether you're looking for a snack, a gourmet dinner, or you're bent on throwing a party, Bill's recipes prove how you can lose the fattening calories without sacrificing taste.

## BASIC MUFFIN MIX

INGREDIENTS

*1 packet Micro Muesli*
*1 teaspoon baking powder*
*½ teaspoon baking soda*
*1 teaspoon cinnamon*
*¼ teaspoon nutmeg*
*⅛ teaspoon mace*
*½ cup whole wheat pastry flour*
*¼ cup egg beaters*
*¾ cup nonfat buttermilk*
*¼ cup skim milk*

GLAZE:

*¼ cup powdered sugar*
*1 tablespoon orange juice*

PROCEDURE

Place all dry ingredients in a bowl and blend. Place all liquids in a separate bowl and blend well. Combine both mixtures and stir just until blended. Spray muffin tin lighly with non-stick vegetable spray. Divide batter evenly into 9 muffins, and bake in 375 degree oven for approximately 15–20 minutes, or until muffins are golden brown, and bounce back to the touch. Glaze muffins as they come out of the oven and then remove from pan.

VARIATIONS:

*Cranberry Orange Muffins*
Add the following ingredients to the basic muffin mix:

*¼ cup orange juice (omit skim milk)*
*½ cup whole cranberries*
*zest of 1 orange*
*⅛ teaspoon nutmeg*

*Apple Cinnamon Muffins*
Add the following ingredients to the basic muffin mix:

*1 Granny Smith apple, peeled, and diced*
*2 tablespoons apple juice concentrate (reduce skim milk in basic mix by 2 tablespoons)*

*Zucchini Carrot Muffins*
Add the following ingredients to the basic muffin mix:

*⅓ cup shredded carrot*
*⅓ cup shredded zucchini*

Basic Muffin Mix
*Per muffin (9 muffins):*

| | |
|---|---|
| Calories – 81 | Fat – 1 gm. |
| Protein – 5 gm. | % of fat – 11% |
| Carbohydrate – 14 gm. | Sodium – 175 mg. |

Cranberry Orange Muffins
*Per muffin (9 muffins):*

| | |
|---|---|
| Calories – 84 | Fat – 1 gm. |
| Protein – 4 gm. | % of fat – 11% |
| Carbohydrate – 15 gm. | Sodium – 172 mg. |

Apple Cinnamon Muffins
*Per muffin (9 muffins):*
Calories – 89
Protein – 4.5 gm.
Carbohydrate – 16 gm.
Fat – 1 gm.
% of fat – 11%
Sodium – 176 mg.

Zucchini-Carrot Muffins
*Per muffin (9 muffins):*
Calories – 83
Protein – 4.7 gm.
Carbohydrate – 14 gm.
Fat – 1 gm.
% of fat – 11%
Sodium – 177 mg.

## GUMBO CHICKEN CREOLE

INGREDIENTS

*1 packet Micro Spanish Rice*
*½ cup diced onion*
*⅓ cup diced green pepper*
*⅓ cup diced celery*
*½ cup diced tomato*
*⅓ cup diced okra*
*¼ teaspoon gumbo file*
*¼ teaspoon thyme*
*1 bay leaf*
*2 oz. cooked chicken*

PROCEDURE

Prepare Spanish Rice as per directions on packet, adding bay leaf. Braise vegetables (cook covered over low heat with small amount of water) until tender. Add thyme and gumbo file. Combine with Spanish Rice. Remove bay leaf before serving.

PER SERVING:
Calories – 453
Protein – 36 gm.
Carbohydrate – 63 gm.
Fat – 7 gm.
% of fat – 14%
Sodium – 844 mg.

# SPAGHETTI SQUASH ITALIENNE
(low-fat recipe)

INGREDIENTS

*1 cup spaghetti squash*
*⅓ cup fresh tomatoes, medium dice*
*⅓ cup onion, large dice*
*⅓ cup mushroom, sliced*
*2 cloves garlic*
*⅓ cup green pepper, large dice*
*⅓ cup eggplant, peeled and diced*
*½ cup tomatoes in juice*
*¼ teaspoon basil*
*¼ teaspoon oregano*
*1 teaspoon Mrs. Dash "garlic and herb"*
*½ teaspoon Parmesan cheese*

PROCEDURE

Cut spaghetti squash in half and remove seeds. Cover bottom of cookie sheet with water and place squash upside-down on pan. Bake in 350 degree oven for 45–60 minutes, or until top of squash is easily pressed down. Saute all vegetables and seasoning in a non-stick saute pan, leaving them a little crisp. Pull squash "meat" away from the skin (it will pull away easily) and warm in a saute pan. Make a ring of hot squash around the center of serving plate and fill the center with vegetable mixture. Sprinkle with Parmesan cheese and serve.

PER SERVING:

| | |
|---|---|
| Calories – 143 | Fat – 1.7 gm. |
| Protein – 5.4 mg. | % of fat – 11% |
| Carbohydrate – 31 gm. | Sodium – 260 mg. |

## CHICKEN CACCIATORE

INGREDIENTS

*1 packet Micro Spanish Rice*
*2 cloves garlic*
*½ cup onion, medium dice*
*¼ teaspoon each basil, oregano, and fennel*
*2 oz. boneless, skinless, cooked chicken breast*
*⅓ cup green pepper, medium dice*
*⅓ cup fresh mushrooms, quartered*
*⅓ cup fresh tomatoes, medium dice*

PROCEDURE

Saute peppers, mushrooms, onions, garlic, and spices together in a non-stick pan until tender. Prepare Spanish Rice as per packet. When ready, combine all ingredients, and serve.

PER SERVING:

| | |
|---|---|
| Calories – 435 | Fat – 7 gm. |
| Protein – 36 gm. | % of fat – 14% |
| Carbohydrate – 58 gm. | Sodium – 799 mg. |

## BANANA-KIWI SMOOTHIE

INGREDIENTS

*1 packet Micro Vanilla Drink mix*
*1 banana*
*1 kiwi*
*½ cup skim milk*
*1 cup ice*
*½ teaspoon vanilla flavoring*
*juice of half a lemon*

PROCEDURE

Pour milk and ice in blender and blend to a slushy consistency. Add vanilla drink mix and fruit and blend on high for 1 minute. Add vanilla flavoring and lemon juice and blend 1 more minute. Serve immediately.

PER SERVING:

| | |
|---|---|
| Calories - 417 | Fat - 3 gm. |
| Protein - 28 gm. | % of fat - 6% |
| Carbohydrate - 74 gm. | Sodium - 568 mg. |

## PINEAPPLE FROSTIE

INGREDIENTS

*1 packet Micro Vanilla Drink mix*
*1 cup fresh pineapple (or canned in juice)*
*½ cup water*
*1 cup ice*
*½ teaspoon vanilla flavoring*

PROCEDURE

Cut fresh pineapple in chunks and whip in blender until light. Add ice and water and blend until ice is crushed. Add vanilla drink mix and vanilla flavoring and blend on high for 1 minute.

PER SERVING:

| | |
|---|---|
| Calories - 294 | Fat - 2.7 gm. |
| Protein - 23 gm. | % of fat - 8% |
| Carbohydrate - 46 gm. | Sodium - 501 mg. |

## BLACK BEAN CHILI DIP WITH BAKED CORN CHIPS

INGREDIENTS
*1 packet Micro Chili*
*2 cups cooked black beans*
*1 tablespoon minced jalapeno peppers*
*1 piece of green onion, diced fine*
*⅓ cup green pepper, finely diced*
*⅓ cup fresh tomatoes, medium diced*
*½ cup nonfat plain yogurt or nonfat sour cream*
*10 corn tortillas*

PROCEDURE

Prepare the chili and let cool. Place the beans, chili, onions, peppers, and tomatoes in a food processor and puree. Place in a crock and chill. When ready to serve, line a large platter with shredded lettuce, and place the crock in the middle of the platter. Cut the corn tortillas in half and cut each half in 5 triangles. Place the corn chips on a cookie sheet and bake in a 300 degree oven until light brown and crisp. Place around the crock of dip and serve.

PER SERVING (6 SERVINGS):

| | |
|---|---|
| Calories – 236 | Fat – 2.4 gm. |
| Protein – 12 gm. | % of fat – 9% |
| Carbohydrate – 43 gm. | Sodium – 225 mg. |

## SPINACH-CHEESE TARRAGON PILLOWS

INGREDIENTS
*1 packet Micro Chicken Tetrazzini*
*1 10 oz. package frozen leaf spinach*
*½ cup onions*
*1 shallot*
*2 cloves garlic*
*1½ cup water or homemade chicken stock*
*Spray vegetable oil*
*Mrs. Dash to taste*
*½ cup ricotta cheese light (Sargento)*
*½ teaspoon tarragon*
*2 tablespoons Parmesan cheese*
*6 sheets phyllo dough*

PROCEDURE

Blanch spinach in water until tender. Spray pan lightly with vegetable oil and saute diced shallots, tarragon, onions, and minced garlic until tender. Add spinach and water or stock and bring to a boil. Turn flame off. Add tetrazzini and let set for 5 minutes (covered). Add ricotta cheese and adjust seasoning. Place a sheet of phyllo dough on counter and spray very lightly with spray oil. Do this a total of 3 times, one layer on top of the other. Cut into 12 equal squares and place one teaspoon of filling in center of square. Fold the dough over the filling then fold the ends under and brush lightly with egg beaters. Sprinkle lightly with Parmesan cheese. Bake in 400 degree oven until golden brown and serve immediately.

PER SERVING:

| | |
|---|---|
| Calories - 961 | Fat - 24 gm. |
| Protein - 60 gm. | % of fat - 22% |
| Carbohydrate - 130 gm. | Sodium - 1658 mg. |

## ARROZO CON POLLO

INGREDIENTS

*1 packet Micro Spanish Rice*
*⅓ cup onion, diced*
*2 cloves garlic*
*⅓ cup fresh tomatoes, medium dice*
*⅓ cup green pepper, medium dice*
*⅛ teaspoon saffron*
*⅓ cup green peas*
*½ cup cooked brown rice*

PROCEDURE

Prepare Spanish rice as per packet, Add saffron, Saute onion, tomato, garlic, and peppers until tender. Heat peas and brown rice and add to Spanish rice. Mix in vegetables and serve.

PER SERVING:

| | |
|---|---|
| Calories - 461 gm. | Fat - 3.5 gm. |
| Protein - 24 gm. | % of fat - 7% |
| Carbohydrate - 85 gm. | Sodium - 813 mg. |

## PINEAPPLE CREAM PIE

INGREDIENTS

*2 Micro Muesli Bars*
*1 packet Micro Vanilla Drink mix*
*1 16 oz. can crushed pineapple (in juice)*
*3 cups pineapple juice*
*7 tablespoons cornstarch*
*5 tablespoons corn syrup*
*4 oz. egg beaters*
*1 teaspoon vanilla extract*
*1 cup Cool Whip Lite*

PROCEDURE

Chop bars in small pieces and warm in microwave for 10 seconds. Press into pie pan. For filling, place pineapple with juice, 1 tablespoon of corn syrup, and ½ cup pineapple juice in saucepan, and bring to a boil. Dissolve 3 tablespoons cornstarch in ½ cup pineapple juice, add to heated pineapple mixture, mix thoroughly, and bring back to a simmer, Pour ⅔ of the filling over the crust and chill, Combine 1¾ cups pineapple juice, 4 tablespoons corn syrup, and vanilla; bring to a boil, Dissolve 4 tablespoons cornstarch in ¼ cup pineapple juice and add to heated mixture, Stir well, bringing back to a boil. Beat in egg beaters, Heat to a simmer, Remove from heat and blend in vanilla shake mix. Pour over pie and cool, When thoroughly cool, spread the remaining pineapple mixture over the top of the pie and then top off with Cool Whip Lite,

PER SERVING (10 SERVINGS):

| | |
|---|---|
| Calories - 216 | Fat - 2.3 gm. |
| Protein - 7 gm. | % of fat - 10% |
| Carbohydrate - 42 gm. | Sodium - 121 mg. |

## SPICY SPANISH RED BEAN SALAD

INGREDIENTS

*2 packets Micro Spanish Rice*
*1 teaspoon diced jalapeno peppers*
*½ cup sliced red onions*
*1 cup cooked red beans*
*1 cup fresh tomatoes, diced*
*Cayenne pepper to taste*
*2 oz. turkey Italian sausage (optional)*

PROCEDURE

Prepare Spanish rice according to packet directions. Meanwhile, bake the sausage and drain any excess grease. Pat the sausage with a paper towel to remove as much of the excess grease as possible. Combine all of the ingredients together and chill for at least 4 hours. Serve on crisp romaine leaves.

PER SERVING (6 SERVINGS):

| | |
|---|---|
| Calories - 134 | Fat - .9 gm. |
| Protein - 8.5 gm. | % of fat - 6% |
| Carbohydrate - 23 gm. | Sodium - 398 mg. |

PER SERVING WITH TURKEY SAUSAGE:

| | |
|---|---|
| Calories - 152 | Fat - 2.2 gm. |
| Protein - 10 gm. | % of fat - 13% |
| Carbohydrate - 23 gm. | Sodium - 475 mg. |

## BRUNSWICK STEW

INGREDIENTS

*1 packet Micro Spanish Rice*
*½ onion, medium dice*
*1 clove garlic, minced*
*¼ cup corn*
*½ cup tomatoes*
*¼ cup Lima beans*
*½ teaspoon liquid smoke*
*2 oz. ground turkey, 97% fat-free (optional)*

PROCEDURE

Combine garlic, onions, corn, and Lima beans. Saute until onions are tender. Meanwhile, prepare Spanish rice according to package. When vegetables are done, add tomatoes, and liquid smoke. Cook ground turkey and drain on paper towel to remove all excess fat. Combine all ingredients and serve.

PER SERVING

| | |
|---|---|
| Calories - 406 | Fat - 3.1 gm. |
| Protein - 23 gm. | % of Fat - 7% |
| Carbohydrate - 74 gm. | Sodium - 890 mg. |

PER SERVING WITH TURKEY:

| | |
|---|---|
| Calories - 514 | Fat - 6.6 gm. |
| Protein - 41 gm. | % of fat - 11% |
| Carbohydrate - 74 gm. | Sodium - 964 mg. |

## BLACK CRAB-STUFFED MUSHROOM CAPS
(low-fat recipe)

INGREDIENTS
*1 dozen jumbo mushroom caps*
*1 stalk green onion, small dice*
*2 shallots, small dice*
*1 cup mushrooms, chopped fine*
*4 oz. imitation crab meat, diced small*
*½ teaspoon sweet vermouth*
*½ teaspoon Mrs. Dash "original"*

PROCEDURE

Remove stems from mushrooms. (Reserve to use in cup of chopped mushrooms.) Lightly coat saute pan with canola oil spray, heat pan, and cook mushroom caps until soft. Set aside. Saute onions, shallots, and mushrooms, adding crab meat when vegetables are almost done. Add vermouth and cook until it evaporates. Place a spoonful of crab filling in each mushroom cap. Bake for 10 minutes in a 350 degree oven.

PER SERVING:

| | |
|---|---|
| Calories - 189 | Fat - 2.5 gm. |
| Protein - 19 gm. | % of fat - 11% |
| Carbohydrate - 26 gm. | Sodium - 958 gm. |

## PEANUT CHIPPER COOKIES

INGREDIENTS
*1 packet Micro Muesli*
*½ Micro Peanut Bar, cut in small pieces*
*⅓ cup flour*
*½ teaspoon baking soda*
*2 oz. egg beaters*
*⅓ cup skim milk*
*1 tablespoon corn syrup*

*PROCEDURE*

Mix all ingredients together and spoon onto a Teflon cookie sheet. Bake in a 350 degree oven until golden brown. (Makes approximately 10 cookies.)

GLAZE

*1 tablespoon unsweetened cocoa*
*1 tablespoon powdered sugar*
*1 teaspoon light corn syrup*
*½ teaspoon skim milk*

Mix all ingredients together and spoon onto cookies.

PER COOKIE:

| | |
|---|---|
| Calories – 74 | Fat – 1 gm. |
| Protein – 3.9 gm. | % of fat – 13% |
| Carbohydrate – 12 gm. | Sodium – 132 mg. |

## CHICKEN FLORENTINE

INGREDIENTS

*1 packet Micro Tetrazzini*
*½ cup sliced mushrooms*
*½ cup onion, medium dice*
*1 shallot, minced*
*½ cup frozen leaf spinach or 1 cup fresh*
*½ teaspoon Parmesan cheese*

PROCEDURE

Spray non-stick saute pan and heat before adding mushrooms, onions, and shallots. Cook until tender, then add spinach and saute on a medium flame for 5 minutes or until the spinach is heated. Meanwhile, prepare tetrazzini as per packet. When spinach mixture is ready, shape it into a ring around the middle of serving plate. Fill center of ring with tetrazzini. Sprinkle with Parmesan cheese and serve.

PER SERVING:

| | |
|---|---|
| Calories – 334 | Fat – 1.9 gm. |
| Protein – 26 gm. | % of fat – 5% |
| Carbohydrate – 55 gm. | Sodium – 945 mg. |

## RASPBERRY MUESLI COOKIES

INGREDIENTS
*1 packet Micro Muesli*
*⅓ cup nonfat buttermilk*
*2 oz. egg beaters*
*2 tablespoons light corn syrup*
*½ cup flour*
*1 tablespoon sugar-free raspberry spread*

GLAZE
*¼ cup powdered sugar*
*1 tablespoon skim milk*
*1 teaspoon sugar-free raspberry spread*

PROCEDURE
Mix the first 6 ingredients together and spoon onto a Teflon cookie sheet. Bake in a 325 degree oven until light brown (approximately 10 minutes). Mix the glaze ingredients together and brush over the baked cookies while warm. Cool and serve.

PER COOKIE (10 COOKIES):

| | |
|---|---|
| Calories - 85 | Fat - .07 gm. |
| Protein - 3.3 gm. | % of fat - 8% |
| Carbohydrate - 16 gm. | Sodium - 72 mg. |

## TEX-MEX POTATO HORS d'OEUVRES

INGREDIENTS
*1 packet Micro Chili*
*12 medium red potatoes*
*Quark (or low-fat sour cream)*
*Nonfat cheddar cheese*

PROCEDURE

Bake potatoes until tender. When done, cut in half right away and scoop out the inside of the potato, keeping a ¼-inch border of potato intact (do this while potato is still hot). Meanwhile, prepare Micro Chili as per directions; time this so the chili is ready when the potatoes are done. Place scooped potato in a bowl and mash into a puree. Combine with prepared chili, and place mixture back into potato shells. (You may spoon this back in if you don't have a pastry bag.) Top with ¼ teaspoon of Quark (or low-fat sour cream if Quark is not available in your area), and sprinkle each potato with ¼ teaspoon of nonfat cheddar cheese. Place under broiler to melt cheese. Serve hot. Makes 24 hors d'oeuvres.

PER HORS D'OEUVRE:

Calories - 66 | Fat - less than 1 gram
Protein - 2.2 gm. | % of fat - less than 1%
Carbohydrate - 14.5 gm. | Sodium - 36.5 mg.

6 SERVINGS (4 HORS D'OEUVRES):

Calories - 264 | Fat - less than 1 gram
Protein - 8.8 gm. | % of fat - 1%
Carbohydrate - 58 gm. | Sodium - 146 mg.

## VEGGIE DIP

INGREDIENTS

*1 packet Micro Chicken Soup*
*½ cup Quark (or low-fat sour cream)*
*½ cup nonfat plain yogurt*
*2 tablespoons shallots, chopped fine*
*1 tablespoon green pepper, chopped fine*
*1 carrot, shredded*

PROCEDURE

Combine all ingredients in bowl and mix well. Chill and serve with fresh veggies for dipping.

VARIATIONS:

*Mexican—add ¼ cup salsa and 2 jalapeno peppers, chopped*
*Pesto—add 1 tablespoon pesto*
*Horseradish—add 1 tablespoon horseradish*

PER SERVING (4 SERVINGS):

Calories–143 | Fat - 1 gm.
Protein–17 gm. | % of fat - 6%
Carbohydrate–15 gm. | Sodium - 312 mg.

Mexican

PER SERVING (4 SERVINGS):

| | |
|---|---|
| Calories - 150 | Fat - 1.3 gm. |
| Protein - 19 gm. | % of fat - 8% |
| Carbohydrate - 17 gm. | Sodium - 492 mg. |

Pesto

PER SERVING (4 SERVINGS):

| | |
|---|---|
| Calories - 164 | Fat - 3 gm. |
| Protein - 19 gm. | % of fat - 17% |
| Carbohydrate - 16 gm. | Sodium - 327 mg. |

Horseradish

PER SERVING (4 SERVINGS):

| | |
|---|---|
| Calories - 144 | Fat - 3 gm. |
| Protein - 19 gm. | % of fat - 17% |
| Carbohydrate - 16 gm. | Sodium - 327 mg. |

## ORANGE FRUIT DIP

INGREDIENTS

*1 packet Micro Orange Drink mix*
*⅓ cup orange juice*
*½ cup nonfat plain yogurt*
*zest of one orange*
*1 orange, peeled and diced*
*3 drops orange flavoring*

PROCEDURE

Combine all ingredients in bowl and mix with wire whisk. Chill and serve over fruit or use as a dip.

PER SERVING (3 SERVINGS):

| | |
|---|---|
| Calories - 124 | Fat - 1 gm. |
| Protein - 10 gm. | % of fat - 6% |
| Carbohydrate - 20 gm. | Sodium - 196 mg. |

# CHEESE STRUDEL

INGREDIENTS

*⅓ cup Sargento Lite Ricotta cheese*
*⅓ cup nonfat cottage cheese*
*1½ oz. nonfat cheddar cheese*
*1½ oz. nonfat mozzarella cheese*
*1½ teaspoons fresh Parmesan cheese*
*6 sheets Phyllo dough (Greek pastry dough)*
*½ of an egg white*

PROCEDURE

Combine all cheeses in a bowl and mix thoroughly. Stack 2 sheets of Phyllo dough and cut into 9 squares. (Repeat with remaining dough.) Place 1 tablespoon of cheese filling in center of each square and brush egg whites on surrounding dough. Fold up into a small square. Place on baking sheet and brush tops with egg whites and a light dusting of Parmesan cheese. Bake in 375 degree oven until pastry is crisp and lightly browned (approx. 15–20 minutes). Serve immediately. Can freeze in raw state and cook as needed.

*Please note:* This recipe doesn't contain a Micro Diet meal. Instead, it is a low-fat choice for dieters who want a recipe on their nondieting days. Cheese Strudel is a wonderful hors d'oeuvre to take to a party.

EACH HORS D'OEUVRE (24 PIECES):

| | |
|---|---|
| Calories – 27 | Fat – .7 gm. |
| Protein – 2.3 gm. | % of fat – 23% |
| Carbohydrate – 2.7 gm. | Sodium – 64 mg. |

## CREAM OF CHICKEN AND SPINACH SOUP

INGREDIENTS

*1 packet Micro Chicken Soup*
*½ cup diced onion*
*⅓ cup diced celery*
*½ cup cooked, chopped spinach*
*¼ teaspoon leaf thyme*
*¼ teaspoon basil*
*1 teaspoon Mrs. Dash*

PROCEDURE

Braise (cook covered on low temperature with a small amount of liquid) onion, celery, and spinach in non-stick pan. Add 1½ cups of water and cook until vegetables are tender. Reserve the water. Prepare Micro soup packet using 1 cup of vegetable water. Add vegetables and spices into soup. Adjust seasoning with Mrs. Dash. Serve immediately.

PER SERVING:

| | |
|---|---|
| Calories - 272 | Fat - 2.5 gm. |
| Protein - 26 gm. | % of fat - 8% |
| Carbohydrate - 40 gm. | Sodium - 975 mg. |

## POTATO LEEK SOUP

INGREDIENTS

*1 packet Micro Chicken Soup*
*1 medium potato, peeled and diced*
*1 leek, diced (use only white portion)*
*½ cup chicken broth*
*½ cup skim milk*
*1 bay leaf*

PROCEDURE

Combine potato, leek, bay leaf, and chicken broth in saucepan. Simmer until vegetables are soft. Drain off liquid and reserve, removing bay leaf. Puree potato and leeks. Heat milk and combine with soup and broth. Add potatoes and leeks, cover for 5–6 minutes. Garnish with chives.

PER SERVING:

| | |
|---|---|
| Calories – 426 | Fat – 3.3 gm. |
| Protein – 32 gm. | % of fat – 7% |
| Carbohydrate – 70 gm. | Sodium – 1321 mg. |

## IN-A-HURRY MICRO CURRY SOUP

INGREDIENTS

*1 packet Micro Chicken Soup*
*⅓ cup diced carrot*
*⅓ cup diced onion*
*⅓ cup diced celery*
*⅓ cup diced apple*
*½ banana, diced*
*1 teaspoon canola oil (optional)*
*½ to 1 teaspoon curry powder*
*8 oz. hot water*

PROCEDURE

Saute all vegetables in oil (or steam, or use non-stick spray). When tender, add curry powder and saute 3 more minutes. Add banana, water, and Micro Chicken Soup. Mix well. Cover 6 minutes. Serve immediately.

PER SERVING:

| | |
|---|---|
| Calories – 329 | Fat – 3 gm. |
| Protein – 24 gm. | % of fat – 8% |
| Carbohydrate – 56 gm. | Sodium – 907 mg. |

PER SERVING WITH OIL:

| | |
|---|---|
| Calories – 369 | Fat – 7 gm. |
| Protein – 24 gm. | % of fat – 17% |
| Carbohydrate – 56 gm. | Sodium – 907 mg. |

## CHICKEN NEWBURG

INGREDIENTS
*1 packet Micro Tetrazzini*
*½ cup onions, medium dice*
*4 shallots, fine dice*
*½ cup mushrooms, quartered*
*½ cup skim milk*
*2 tablespoons cooking sherry (optional)*
*2 oz. cooked chicken (optional)*
*¼ teaspoon paprika*

PROCEDURE
Prepare tetrazzini with ½ cup skim milk and ½ cup water. Using non-stick spray, saute onions, shallots, mushrooms, and paprika for 2 minutes. Add cooking sherry, if desired, and continue to cook until sherry has almost cooked away. When tetrazzini is ready, combine with vegetable mixture, and serve immediately.

PER SERVING:

| | |
|---|---|
| Calories – 369 | Fat – 1.7 gm. |
| Protein – 28 gm. | % of fat – 4% |
| Carbohydrate – 61 gm. | Sodium – 910 mg. |

PER SERVING WITH SHERRY AND CHICKEN:

| | |
|---|---|
| Calories – 502 | Fat – 3.7 gm. |
| Protein – 46 gm. | % of fat – 7% |
| Carbohydrate – 64 gm. | Sodium – 953 mg. |

## TETRAZZINI ASPARAGUS CREPES

CREPES–INGREDIENTS
*½ cup whole-wheat pastry flour*
*½ cup water*
*2 egg whites*
*1 teaspoon Butter Buds*

CREPES–PROCEDURE

Combine all ingredients in a bowl and mix thoroughly with a wire whisk. Spray a 6–8 inch non-stick skillet with vegetable spray (spray one time only). Heat skillet. Ladle in 2 tablespoons of batter and swirl to cover bottom of pan. Brown both sides. Continue until all batter is used. Crepes should be thin. Unused crepes may be wrapped with waxed paper in between each one and frozen for future use.

PER CREPE (MAKES 12):

| | |
|---|---|
| Calories – 21 | Fat – .2 gm |
| Protein – 1.3 gm | Sodium – 20 mg |
| Carbohydrate – 3.9 gm | |

FILLING-INGREDIENTS

*1 packet Micro Tetrazzini*
*¼ cup zucchini*
*¼ cup yellow squash*
*½ cup onion*
*⅓ cup mushrooms*
*1 shallot*
*2 tablespoons nonfat mozzarella cheese*
*Fresh asparagus*
*½ teaspoon canola oil (optional)*

FILLING-PROCEDURE

Cut squash into matchlike strips, cut onion into small dice, mince shallot, and slice mushrooms. Place all vegetables (except asparagus) in hot skillet with oil and saute until tender.* While vegetables are cooking, blanch asparagus in boiling water, and make Micro Tetrazzini. Combine tetrazzini with vegetable medley.

TO ASSEMBLE

Place asparagus (2 small spears or one large) in middle of each crepe. Top with ⅓ of tetrazzini mixture. Roll up crepes and place seam-side-down on serving plate. Sprinkle nonfat mozzarella cheese over stuffed crepes and place under broiler until cheese melts.

*you may steam or blanch

PER SERVING (2 SERVINGS OF 3 CREPES):

| | |
|---|---|
| Calories – 286 | Fat – 1.6 gm |
| Protein – 25 gm | % of fat – 5% |
| Carbohydrate – 46 gm | Sodium – 642 mg |

WITH OIL:

| | |
|---|---|
| Calories – 297 | Fat – 2.7 gm |
| Protein – 25 gm | % of fat – 8% |
| Carbohydrate – 46 gm | Sodium – 642 mg |

# SPAGHETTI SQUASH ALFREDO

INGREDIENTS

*1 packet Micro Tetrazzini*
*1 cup spaghetti squash*
*fresh garlic*
*½ teaspoon canola oil (optional)*
*½ cup yellow squash*
*½ cup zucchini*
*½ cup mushrooms*
*2 cloves garlic*
*½ teaspoon canola oil (optional)*

PROCEDURE

Cut spaghetti squash in half lengthwise. Place on a cookie sheet, cut side down, with water. Bake in oven at 350 degrees until squash indents when pressed (approximately 45 minutes–1 hour).

Cut yellow squash and zucchini in small strips (julienne style), slice mushrooms, and mince garlic, and saute all in oil* in saute pan until tender. Prepare Micro Tetrazzini, using ½ cup water and ½ cup skim milk.

Remove spaghetti squash from shell and saute with 1 clove minced garlic in ½ teaspoon oil.* Cook until warmed.

To arrange, place spaghetti squash on plate in a ring. Fill the ring with Micro Tetrazzini and top tetrazzini with sauteed vegetables. Sprinkle with Parmesan cheese and serve hot.

* may steam or use non-stick spray

PER SERVING:

| | |
|---|---|
| Calories – 411 | Fat – 2.8 gm |
| Protein – 30 mg | % of fat – 6% |
| Carbohydrate – 69 mg | Sodium – 949 mg |

WITH OIL:

| | |
|---|---|
| Calories – 452 | Fat – 7.3 gm |
| Protein – 30 mg | % of fat – 14% |
| Carbohydrate – 69 mg | Sodium – 949 mg |

# CHICKEN POT PIE

INGREDIENTS

*1 packet Micro Tetrazzini*
*½ cup onions, large dice*
*⅓ cup celery, large dice*
*⅓ cup carrots, large dice*
*⅓ cup potato, medium dice*
*1 teaspoon chopped parsley*
*1½ cups water*
*4 sheets Phyllo dough (Greek pastry dough)*
*1 tablespoon egg beaters*
*1 teaspoon Mrs. Dash*

PROCEDURE

Place onions, celery, carrots, and potatoes in pot with 1½ cups water and bring to a boil. Simmer for 10 minutes. Strain water off of vegetables and use 1¼ cups of liquid to prepare Tetrazzini. When Tetrazzini is done, combine with vegetables. Meanwhile, stack 4 sheets of Phyllo dough together and place on a Teflon cookie sheet. Brush with egg beaters and bake in 350 degree oven until light brown and crisp. Pour Tetrazzini mixture in bottom of an 8 x 8 baking dish. Place cooked Phyllo dough on top of mixture and serve immediately.

PER SERVING (2 SERVINGS):

| | |
|---|---|
| Calories – 302 | Fat – 3.7 gm |
| Protein – 16 gm | % of fat – 11% |
| Carbohydrate – 51 gm | Sodium – 535 mg |

## MEDLEY BAKED STUFFED POTATO

INGREDIENTS

*1 packet Micro Tetrazzini*
*1 medium baking potato*
*¼ cup broccoli, medium dice*
*¼ cup onion, diced*
*¼ cup mushrooms, sliced*
*1 oz. nonfat cheddar cheese*

PROCEDURE

While potato is baking, steam broccoli, onions, and mushrooms until tender. When potato is almost done, prepare Tetrazzini as per directions on the package. Cut a slice off of the long side of the potato large enough to allow you to scoop the potato out of the shell, leaving enough next to the skin to keep shell intact. Mix scooped potato and nonfat cheddar cheese into Tetrazzini, making a thick "paste" type mixture, and spoon back into potato shell. Top with steamed vegetables and serve immediately.

PER SERVING:

Calories – 550
Protein – 36 gm
Carbohydrate – 98 gm
Fat – 1.5 gm
% of fat – 2%
Sodium – 1155 mg

## CHICKEN MUSHROOM STRUDEL

INGREDIENTS

*1 packet Micro Tetrazzini*
*6 sheets Phyllo dough (Greek pastry dough)*
*2 cups sliced mushrooms*
*½ cup onions, fine dice*
*2 shallots, fine dice*
*2 cloves garlic, minced*
*½ teaspoon basil*
*3 oz. nonfat mozzarella cheese*
*⅓ cup white wine (optional)*
*2 oz. cooked chicken*
*1 teaspoon Parmesan cheese*

PROCEDURE

Spray saute pan with vegetable spray and cook mushrooms, onions, shallots, and garlic until tender. Add white wine, if desired, and basil, and cook until wine has evaporated. Meanwhile, prepare Tetrazzini as per directions on package. To assemble, place all 6 sheets of Phyllo dough together on cutting board. Spread Tetrazzini along long edge of dough, 4″ from the bottom (leave enough space at either end to tuck under). Top with vegetable mixture and then cheese. Roll strudel by bringing bottom edge up over the filling and continue to roll to the top of the dough. Fold under the ends and press down gently to slightly flatten. Place on baking sheet (spray with vegetable spray), brush lightly with egg beaters, sprinkle 1 teaspoon Parmesan cheese over the top, and bake in 350 degree oven for approximately 25–30 minutes, or until dough is crisp and golden brown. Serve immediately.

PER SERVING (2 SERVINGS):

| | |
|---|---|
| Calories – 462 | Fat – 6.4 gm |
| Protein – 41 gm | % of fat – 13% |
| Carbohydrate – 59 gm | Sodium – 1000 mg |

WITH WINE:

| | |
|---|---|
| Calories – 488 | Fat – 6.4 gm |
| Protein – 41 gm | % of fat – 12% |
| Carbohydrate – 59 gm | Sodium – 1023 mg |

## CHICKEN VERONIQUE

INGREDIENTS

*1 packet Micro Tetrazzini*
*12 white grapes*
*½ cup onions, minced*
*2 shallots, minced*
*⅓ cup carrots, cut in matchlike strips*
*⅓ cup mushrooms, sliced*
*2 oz. cooked chicken (optional)*
*¼ teaspoon thyme*

PROCEDURE

Place grapes in water, bring to a boil, and cook for 2 minutes. Remove with slotted spoon. Using a non-stick saute pan and vegetable spray, saute vegetables and thyme until vegetables are tender. Meanwhile, prepare Tetrazzini as per directions on packet. When ready, combine all ingredients, and serve immediately.

PER SERVING:

| | |
|---|---|
| Calories – 382 | Fat – 1.7 gm |
| Protein – 24 gm | % of fat – 4% |
| Carbohydrate – 71 gm | Sodium – 859 mg |

WITH CHICKEN:

| | |
|---|---|
| Calories – 475 | Fat – 3.8 gm |
| Protein – 42 gm | % of fat – 7% |
| Carbohydrate – 71 gm | Sodium – 901 mg |

# CHICKEN DIJON

INGREDIENTS

*1 packet Micro Tetrazzini*
*1 shallot, diced fine*
*½ cup onion, diced*
*½ cup sliced mushrooms*
*½ teaspoon canola oil (optional)*
*¼ teaspoon rosemary*
*¼ teaspoon tarragon*
*1 teaspoon Dijon mustard*
*1 teaspoon Parmesan cheese*
*2 oz. skinless, boneless baked chicken (optional)*

PROCEDURE

Combine vegetables, rosemary, and tarragon and saute in canola oil* until tender. While vegetables are cooking, prepare Tetrazzini as per directions, adding ¼ cup more water than package calls for. When Tetrazzini is ready, combine all ingredients, and mix thoroughly.

*may steam or use non-stick spray

PER SERVING:

| | |
|---|---|
| Calories – 320 | Fat – 2.2 gm |
| Protein – 24 gm | % of fat – 6% |
| Carbohydrate – 51 gm | Sodium – 948 mg |

WITH CHICKEN AND OIL:

| | |
|---|---|
| Calories – 433 | Fat – 6.5 gm |
| Protein – 42 gm | % of fat – 14% |
| Carbohydrate – 51 gm | Sodium – 948 mg |

# CHICKEN DIVAN

INGREDIENTS

*1 packet Micro Tetrazzini*
*½ cup cooked brown rice*
*1 cup broccoli fleurettes*
*⅓ cup onion, small dice*
*2 shallots*
*⅓ cup mushrooms, quartered*
*1 teaspoon Parmesan cheese*
*1 teaspoon chopped parsley*
*¼ teaspoon marjoram*
*2 oz. cooked chicken (optional)*

PROCEDURE

Prepare brown rice according to directions on box. Meanwhile, prepare Tetrazzini according to packet, steam broccoli until tender, and saute remaining vegetables and marjoram in non-stick pan (using vegetable spray) until tender. Arrange cooked rice in a ring on serving plate. Place broccoli in center of ring, pour on Tetrazzini, and top with Parmesan cheese and chopped parsley.

PER SERVING:

Calories – 462
Protein – 31 gm
Carbohydrate – 81 gm
Fat – 3.2 gm
% of fat – 6%
Sodium – 904 mg

WITH CHICKEN:

Calories – 556
Protein – 48 gm
Carbohydrate – 81 gm
Fat – 5.2 gm
% of fat – 8%
Sodium – 945 mg

## CHILI-STUFFED PEPPER

INGREDIENTS

*1 packet Micro Chili*
*2 oz. ground turkey (97% fat free)*
*½ cup onions, diced*
*2 cloves garlic, minced*
*½ cup mushrooms, sliced*
*½ cup tomatoes, diced*
*1 piece green onion, diced*
*1 large green pepper*
*½ teaspoon chili powder*
*¼ teaspoon cumin*

PROCEDURE

Trim top off of green pepper. Place whole pepper in boiling water for 5–7 minutes, or until tender but still firm. Saute turkey, onions, garlic, tomatoes, green onion, mushrooms, top of green pepper (chopped), chili powder, and cumin in non-stick pan until turkey is completely cooked and vegetables are tender. Meanwhile, prepare chili as per directions on package. Combine chili and vegetable mixture and spoon into green pepper. Sprinkle a small amount of nonfat cheddar cheese over the top and place under broiler until cheese is melted. Serve immediately.

PER SERVING:

| | |
|---|---|
| Calories – 430 | Fat – 8.9 gm |
| Protein – 34 gm | % of fat – 18% |
| Carbohydrate – 59 gm | Sodium – 700 mg |

## CHICKEN JARDINIERE

INGREDIENTS

*1 packet Micro Diet Tetrazzini*
*¼ cup green onion, diced*
*¼ cup yellow squash, cut in small strips*
*¼ cup zucchini, cut in small strips*
*¼ cup tomatoes, diced*
*¼ cup mushrooms, sliced*
*¼ cup snow peas, whole*
*¼ cup carrots, cut in small strips*
*¼ teaspoon thyme*

PROCEDURE

Spray non-stick saute pan with vegetable spray, add vegetables and thyme and saute until tender. Meanwhile, prepare Tetrazzini as per directions on package. Using cooked vegetables, make ring in center of serving plate and fill with Tetrazzini. Serve immediately.

PER SERVING:

| | |
|---|---|
| Calories – 321 | Fat – 1.6 gm |
| Protein – 24 gm | % of fat – 4% |
| Carbohydrate – 54 gm | Sodium – 858 mg |

## VEGETABLE PITA PIZZA

INGREDIENTS

*¼ cup mushrooms, sliced*
*¼ cup onions, small dice*
*¼ cup peppers, small dice*
*¼ cup tomatoes, small dice*
*1 piece whole wheat pita bread*
*4 tablespoons pizza sauce*
*1½ oz. nonfat mozzarella cheese*

PROCEDURE

Steam vegetables until tender. Place pita bread on cookie sheet and spread with half of pizza sauce. Top with cooked vegetables followed by cheese and then remaining sauce. Sprinkle lightly with Parmesan cheese and bake in 375 degree oven until hot and cheese is browned. Serve immediately.

*Please note:* This recipe does not include a Micro Diet item. It is, however, a good menu selection for dieters who desire a very low-fat meal.

PER SERVING:

| | |
|---|---|
| Calories – 245 | Fat – 3 gm |
| Protein – 20 gm | % of fat – 11% |
| Carbohydrate – 35 gm | Sodium – 1053 mg |

## CHOCOLATE MOUSSE PIE

INGREDIENTS

*1 packet Chocolate Micro Drink*
*2 Chocolate Micro Bars*
*½ cup skim milk*
*3 tablespoons dry unsweetened cocoa*
*½ teaspoon almond flavoring*
*1 teaspoon chocolate flavoring*
*1 teaspoon vanilla flavoring*
*2 egg whites*
*2 tablespoons powdered sugar*
*½ teaspoon cream of tartar*
*1 packet unflavored gelatin*
*¼ cup cold water*

PROCEDURE

Crush Micro bars with rolling pin and place in bottom of serving dish. Chill. Whip egg whites and cream of tartar together until frothy. Add powdered sugar and whip until stiff. Set aside. Dissolve gelatin in cold water. Let set for 2 minutes. In blender, combine milk, cocoa, and Micro Chocolate Drink mix and blend 1 minute. Add flavorings and 6 ice cubes. Blend 1 minute. Place gelatin mixture on low flame and bring to a simmer. Slowly pour hot liquid in a steady stream into drink mixture (blend as you pour). Let mixture begin to set in fridge. Fold in egg white mixture and pour over Micro bar "crust." Chill until firm.

PER SERVING (8 SERVINGS):

| | |
|---|---|
| Calories - 125 | Fat - 3 gm |
| Protein - 9 gm | % of fat - 20% |
| Carbohydrate - 17 gm | Sodium - 110 mg |

## MUESLI CHEESE STRUDEL

INGREDIENTS

*1 packet Micro Muesli*
*6 sheets Phyllo dough*
*⅛ cup egg beaters (for brushing dough)*
*½ Granny Smith apple, chopped*
*⅛ cup Sargento Light Ricotta Cheese*
*⅛ cup nonfat cottage cheese*
*⅛ cup Quark (may substitute cottage or ricotta cheese)*

*1 teaspoon cinnamon*
*¼ cup raisins*

GLAZE:
*1 tablespoon powdered sugar*
*1 teaspoon water*

PROCEDURE

Combine chopped apple, cheeses, cinnamon, and raisins in a bowl and mix thoroughly. Place 1 sheet of Phyllo dough on a cutting board. (This dough is very fragile. Always keep unused portion covered with a towel to keep it from drying out.) Using a pastry brush, lightly brush with egg beaters, leaving as light a coating as possible. Place a second sheet of Phyllo dough directly on top of the first one and continue the brushing/layering process until all the dough is used. Sprinkle a package of Muesli over the top layer of brushed dough. Spoon filling onto Phyllo dough starting 4″ from the bottom of the long side of the dough, creating a 3″ strip of filling (be sure to leave enough space at either end to tuck under). Roll the strudel by bringing the bottom edge up over the filling and continue to roll all the way to the top edge. Fold under the ends. Gently press down on the top of the strudel to flatten it slightly. Place on a baking sheet (spray with vegetable spray), brush lightly with egg beaters, and bake in 375 degree oven for approximately 20–25 minutes, or until the dough is golden brown and very crisp. As soon as you remove it from the oven, brush top with sugar glaze. Let cool slightly and serve.

PER SERVING (3 SERVINGS):

| | |
|---|---|
| Calories – 310 | Fat – 5.5 gm |
| Protein – 16 gm | % of fat – 16% |
| Carbohydrate – 50 gm | Sodium – 316 mg |

## RASPBERRY CHEESE STRUDEL

INGREDIENTS

*1 packet Micro Vanilla Drink*
*6 sheets phyllo dough*
*⅛ cup Sargento Lite Ricotta Cheese*
*⅛ cup nonfat cottage cheese*
*⅛ cup Quark (may substitute cottage or ricotta cheese)*
*⅛ cup nonfat plain yogurt*
*1 tablespoon egg beaters (mix into cheese and raspberry combination)*
*½ cup raspberries*
*1 tablespoon powdered sugar*
*1 oz. egg beaters (brush onto dough before baking)*

GLAZE:

*1 tablespoon powdered sugar*
*1 teaspoon water*

PROCEDURE

Combine cheeses, yogurt, egg beaters, and powdered sugar and mix. Add in Vanilla Drink mix in its powdered state and mix thoroughly. Gently fold in raspberries. Set filling aside and refer to Muesli Cheese Strudel (previous recipe) for strudel assembly instructions (important: Omit Muesli).

PER SERVING (3 SERVINGS):

Calories – 271
Protein – 19 gm
Carbohydrate – 38 gm
Fat – 5 gm
% of fat – 17%
Sodium – 331 mg

## CHOCOLATE MOUSSE

INGREDIENTS

*1 packet Micro Chocolate Drink*
*2 tablespoons unsweetened cocoa*
*¼ package chocolate fudge pudding mix (sugar-free)*
*3 tablespoons skim milk*
*1 cup Cool Whip Lite*

PROCEDURE

Mix chocolate drink, cocoa, pudding, and skim milk into a paste. Fold the Cool Whip into the paste and place in cups to chill before serving.

PER SERVING (2 SERVINGS):

| | |
|---|---|
| Calories - 214 | Fat - 6.5 gm |
| Protein - 13 gm | % of fat - 26% |
| Carbohydrate - 29 gm | Sodium - 397 mg |

## CHOCOLATE MINT PIE

INGREDIENTS

*1 packet Micro Vanilla Drink*
*1 packet Micro Chocolate Drink*
*2 Micro Chocolate Bars*
*1 package vanilla instant pudding mix (nonfat and sugar-free)*
*1 package chocolate instant pudding mix (nonfat and sugar-free)*
*2 tablespoons unsweetened cocoa powder*
*mint flavoring*
*1 cup Cool Whip Lite*

PROCEDURE

Cut chocolate bars into small pieces and warm in microwave for 10 seconds. Press into bottom of pie pan and refrigerate. Combine vanilla pudding powder and vanilla drink mix. Follow directions on pudding mix, using skim milk. Add ⅛ teaspoon mint flavoring (and green food coloring if you wish). Pour on top of chocolate crust and let set in refrigerator. Combine chocolate fudge pudding powder, and chocolate drink mix, and cocoa and follow directions on pudding mix, using skim milk. Add ⅛ teaspoon mint flavoring and let set. Spoon over top of vanilla layer and let set in refrigerator. When firm, spread 1 cup of Cool Whip Lite over the top. Refrigerater for 2 hours before serving.

PER SERVING (8 SERVINGS):

| | |
|---|---|
| Calories - 218 | Fat - 4.7 gm |
| Protein - 14 gm | % of fat - 19% |
| Carbohydrate - 32 gm | Sodium - 538 mg |

## LOW-FAT PARTY MIX

INGREDIENTS

*1 Micro Muesli Bar*
*1 Micro Peanut Bar*
*1 cup air-popped popcorn, lightly chopped*
*1 cup nonfat pretzels, slightly crushed*
*1 cup raisins*
*1 cup mini honey-nut rice cakes*
*Molly McButter*

PROCEDURE

Make the popcorn and chop slightly with a knife. Place the pretzels in your hand and crush slightly. Cut the bars and rice cakes into small pieces. Combine all the ingredients. Mix and serve.

PER SERVING (6 SERVINGS):

| | |
|---|---|
| Calories - 210 | Fat - 2.3 gm |
| Protein - 7 gm | % of fat - 10% |
| Carbohydrate - 43 gm | Sodium - 228 mg |

## HOT CRAB DIP
(low-fat recipe)

INGREDIENTS

*4 oz. imitation crab meat*
*4 oz. nonfat mayonnaise*
*4 oz. sliced mushrooms*
*2 stalks green onions*
*4 oz. nonfat Quark, or cottage cheese, or ricotta cheese*
*2 oz. nonfat mozzarella cheese*
*2 shallots*
*6 pieces whole wheat pita bread*
*1 oz. Parmesan cheese*

PROCEDURE

Slice the pita bread open into two flat pieces. Cut each piece in half, and then cut each half into 5 triangles, and place on a cookie sheet. Bake in a 325 degree oven until slightly brown and crisp. Dice the shallots and green onions and saute in a non-stick saute pan with a quick spray of canola oil until tender. Add the crab and heat. Combine all the ingredients except the pita bread. Place mixture in a Pyrex baking dish and sprinkle with Parmesan cheese. Bake in a 350 degree oven for 30 minutes. Serve with the toasted pita chips.

PER SERVING (6 SERVINGS):

| | |
|---|---|
| Calories - 225 | Fat - 2.5 gm |
| Protein - 18 gm | % of fat - 10% |
| Carbohydrate - 31 gm | Sodium - 865 mg |

# MUESLI PANCAKES

INGREDIENTS

*1 packet Micro Muesli*
*1 tablespoon raspberry sugar-free spread*
*2 tablespoons light corn syrup*
*⅓ cup nonfat buttermilk*
*½ teaspoon baking soda*
*½ cup flour*
*2 oz. egg beaters*

PROCEDURE

Place the Muesli, baking soda, and flour in a bowl. In a separate bowl, mix the remaining ingredients. Combine the two mixtures and stir until well blended. Spoon the mixture onto a heated griddle on low heat and brown on both sides. Serve with powdered sugar or a small amount of sugar-free syrup.

PER PANCAKE (10 PANCAKES):

| | |
|---|---|
| Calories - 73 | Fat - .7 gm |
| Protein - 3.3 gm | % of fat - 9% |
| Carbohydrate - 13 gm | Sodium - 113 mg |

## CHILI FAJITA

INGREDIENTS

*1 packet Micro Chili*
*¼ teaspoon cumin*
*2 cloves garlic, minced*
*2 oz. white meat chicken, cut in strips*
*½ cup onion, sliced*
*1 teaspoon Worcestershire sauce*
*1 stalk green onion*
*¼ cup nonfat Quark, nonfat sour cream, or nonfat plain yogurt*
*1 large flour tortilla (check the nutritional information on the package because some brands are higher in fat than others)*
*½ cup shredded lettuce*

PROCEDURE

Prepare Micro Chili as per packet directions. Combine onions, garlic, and cumin and saute in non-stick pan until tender. Mix Worcestershire sauce with chicken. Let set for 2 minutes and then combine with onions and cook until chicken is done. Add chili to chicken mixture and place on tortilla. Top with diced green onion, lettuce, and Quark. Roll up and serve!

PER SERVING:

| | |
|---|---|
| Calories – 568 | Fat – 5.4 gm |
| Protein – 59 gm | % of fat – 8% |
| Carbohydrate – 73 gm | Sodium – 840 mg |

## SHRIMP ETOUFFE

INGREDIENTS

*1 packet Micro Spanish Rice*
*¼ teaspoon basil*
*¼ teaspoon thyme*
*¼ teaspoon Mrs. Dash "Garlic and Seasoning"*
*½ cup diced onions*
*⅓ cup diced celery*
*⅓ cup diced green pepper*
*⅓ cup diced green onion*
*⅓ cup V-8 juice*
*2 teaspoons cornstarch*
*¼ cup water (cold)*
*2 oz. cooked peeled shrimp (diced small)*

PROCEDURE

Saute the vegetables and diced shrimp in a non-stick saute pan until tender, adding spices when veggies are almost done. Meanwhile, prepare Spanish rice as per directions. Next add the V-8 juice to the veg./shrimp mixture and bring to a boil. Dissolve cornstarch in water and add to the mixture. Stir well and bring back to a simmer. Combine with Spanish rice and serve.

PER SERVING:

| | |
|---|---|
| Calories - 412 | Fat - 3.3 gm |
| Protein - 31 gm | % of fat - 7% |
| Carbohydrate - 64 gm | Sodium - 118 mg |

## CHILI CHEESE PUFFS

INGREDIENTS

*1 packet Micro Chili*
*¼ cup green onion, diced very small*
*½ teaspoon fat-free cheddar cheese*
*¼ teaspoon fat-free sour cream*
*6 sheets Phyllo dough*
*Spray oil*

PROCEDURE

Prepare Micro Chili as per directions on packet. Cool slightly. Place one sheet of Phyllo dough on cutting board and coat very lightly with spray oil. Place second sheet directly on top of first and cut into 6 squares. Put a small spoonful of chili in center of square and top with small amount of diced onion, ½ tsp nonfat cheddar cheese and ¼ tsp nonfat sour cream. Fold dough into a small square, being sure to encase off of the filling. Place fold-side-down on baking sheet. Repeat process with remaining 4 sheets of Phyllo dough. Bake in 375° oven for approximately 10 minutes or until golden. Makes 18 hors d'oeuvres.

PER HORS D'OEUVRE:

| | |
|---|---|
| Calories - 36 | Fat - .7 gm |
| Protein - 2 gm | % of fat - 18% |
| Carbohydrate - 5.4 gm | Sodium - 61 mg |

## MOCK GUACAMOLE

INGREDIENTS

*2 cups cooked green split peas*
*1 packet Micro Pea Soup*
*3 Roma tomatoes*
*2 pieces green onion*
*2 cloves garlic*
*2 tablespoons jalapeno peppers*
*½ cup salsa*
*1 teaspoon lemon juice*

PROCEDURE

Cook one package of green split dried peas according to directions (cook until thick). Prepare Micro Pea Soup according to package. Combine cooked peas, and pea soup, and puree. Cool. Cut tomatoes, onion, and jalapeno peppers into small dice. Mince garlic and mix with salsa. Combine all ingredients, mix well, chill, and serve. Makes 2 cups.

(For dipping, look for baked [not fried] corn chips in the nutrition area of your supermarket, or make your own nonfat chips by cutting pita bread into small triangles and baking in 300° oven until crisp.)

PER SERVING:

| | |
|---|---|
| Calories – 779 | Fat – 10 gm |
| Protein – 50 gm | % of fat – 11% |
| Carbohydrate – 132 gm | Sodium – 1439 mg |

## CHOCOLATE-PEANUT BUTTER CRUNCH PIE

INGREDIENTS

*1 Micro Crunchy Peanut Bar*
*2 Micro Peanut Bars*
*1 packet Micro Chocolate Drink*
*1 package sugar-free, fat-free instant chocolate pudding mix*
*Skim milk (as per the amount called for on pudding mix box)*
*1½ cup Cool Whip Lite*

PROCEDURE

Dice two Micro Peanut Bars and press into bottom of pie pan. Combine dry pudding mix and Micro Chocolate Drink mix and add in skim milk to prepare filling. Pour over crust and refrigerate until filling sets. Spread Cool Whip over top of pie. Chop Micro Crunchy Peanut Bar into small pieces and sprinkle over top. Cut into 10 slices and serve. Serves 10.

PER SERVING:

| | |
|---|---|
| Calories - 154 | Fat - 4.1 gm |
| Protein - 9 gm | % of fat - 23% |
| Carbohydrate - 22 gm | Sodium - 323 mg |

## LAYERED SALAD

INGREDIENTS

*½ head lettuce*
*1 cucumber, peeled*
*3 carrots*
*½ pound mushrooms*
*1 can kidney beans*
*2 large tomatoes, sliced*
*3 yellow squash*
*2 packets Micro Spanish Rice*
*1 cup nonfat ranch dressing*

PROCEDURE

Shred lettuce and carrot; slice tomatoes, cucumbers, and mushrooms (slice thin). Cut squash into ¼″ thick slices. Prepare Micro Spanish rice as per directions on package. Place half of lettuce on bottom of clear glass straight-sided salad serving bowl. Layer the vegetables as they are listed. Place layers of ranch dressing and Spanish rice alternately with the vegetables. Keep layering until all the veggies, rice, and dressing are used up. Refrigerate until well chilled and serve. (Serves 6)

PER SERVING (6 SERVINGS):

| | |
|---|---|
| Calories - 260 | Fat - 1.6 gm. |
| Protein - 13 gm | % of fat - 5% |
| Carbohydrate - 50 gm. | Sodium - 943 mg. |

## GAZPACHO

INGREDIENTS

*½ medium onion, small dice*
*½ green pepper, small dice*
*1 cucumber, peeled and diced*
*1 clove garlic, minced*
*3 Roma tomatoes, cored and diced*
*1 carrot, shredded*
*2 packets Micro Spanish Rice*
*1 packet Micro Tomato Soup*

PROCEDURE

Prepare Micro Spanish Rice and Tomato Soup as per directions on package. Combine, set aside, and let cool. Chop vegetables. Combine all ingredients, mix well, and refrigerate. Serve cold. (Serves 4)

PER SERVING:

| | |
|---|---|
| Calories - 240 | Fat - 2.5 gm |
| Protein - 15 gm | % of fat - 9% |
| Carbohydrate - 41 gm | Sodium - 567 mg |

## STUFFED MANICOTTI

INGREDIENTS

*1 packet Micro Tetrazzini*
*⅓ cup frozen leaf spinach, thawed, and drained*
*⅓ cup diced onions*
*½ cup sliced mushrooms*
*4 cooked manicotti shells*
*1 cup nonfat ricotta cheese*
*½ cup nonfat mozzarella cheese*
*2 teaspoons Parmesan cheese*
*4 slices fresh tomato*
*1 tablespoon fresh basil*

PROCEDURE

Cook manicotti shells according to box directions. Prepare one package of Micro Tetrazzini according to the package. Saute spinach, onions, and mushrooms together until onions are transparent. Combine with ricotta cheese, mozzarella cheese, and Tetrazzini. Stuff the manicotti shells. Place 2 shells together and top with two slices of tomato and half of the fresh basil. Sprinkle with Parmesan cheese. Repeat process with remaining two shells and place in a baking dish. Bake for ten minutes in 375° oven. (Serves 2)

PER SERVING:

| | |
|---|---|
| Calories - 561 | Fat - 17 gm |
| Protein - 40 gm | % of fat - 27% |
| Carbohydrate - 62 gm | Sodium - 781 mg |

## SPANISH RICE AND COUSCOUS SALAD

INGREDIENTS

*2 teaspoons yellow mustard*
*¼ cup balsamic vinegar*
*2 cloves garlic*
*2 pieces green onion*
*½ cup sliced mushrooms*
*¼ cup diced onions*
*2 cup couscous cooked*
*2 packets Micro Spanish Rice*

PROCEDURE

Prepare couscous as per directions on the box. Make Micro Spanish Rice according to packet. Combine all ingredients, mix well, and refrigerate at least 4 hours before serving. (Serves 4)

PER SERVING:

| | |
|---|---|
| Calories - 241 | Fat - 1.3 gm |
| Protein - 12 gm | % of fat - 5% |
| Carbohydrate - 45 gm | Sodium - 413 mg |

## SPICY SHRIMP ROLL-UPS

INGREDIENTS

*8 oz. cooked shrimp, peeled and deveined*
*½ cup sliced onions*
*2 cloves garlic*
*2 Roma tomatoes*
*⅓ cup sliced mushrooms*
*4 flour tortillas*
*½ cup shredded lettuce*
*3 tablespoons nonfat plain yogurt*
*2 teaspoon diced jalapeno peppers*
*1 packet Micro Spanish Rice*

PROCEDURE

Prepare shrimp and set aside. Saute onions, garlic, diced fresh tomatoes, and mushrooms in a non-stick pan until tender. Prepare Micro Spanish Rice according to the directions on the package. Spread flour tortillas with yogurt and top with lettuce. Combine all other ingredients together, mix well, and divide over the tortillas. Roll up tortillas and serve 2 per person.

PER SERVING:

| | |
|---|---|
| Calories - 491 | Fat - 6.3 gm |
| Protein - 41 gm | % of fat - 12% |
| Carbohydrate - 68 gm | Sodium - 700 mg |

## MANHATTAN CLAM CHOWDER

INGREDIENTS

*1 can chopped clams*
*1 small bottle clam juice*
*1 cup water*
*2 packets Micro Spanish Rice*
*1 onion, medium dice*
*2 stalks celery, medium dice*
*1 green pepper, medium dice*
*1 peeled Idaho potato, medium dice*
*1 teaspoon thyme*
*1 bay leaf*
*1 teaspoon Mrs. Dash "Onions & Spice"*

PROCEDURE

Combine all ingredients except Spanish rice in saucepan and simmer until all vegetables are tender. Prepare Micro Spanish Rice as per packet, but use only ½ the amount of water called for. Combine soup with other ingredients, mix well, and serve while hot. (Serves 2)

PER SERVING:

| | |
|---|---|
| Calories - 395 | Fat - 3.5 gm |
| Protein - 27 gm | % of fat - 8% |
| Carbohydrate - 66 gm | Sodium - 842 mg |

## CREAM OF ASPARAGUS SOUP

INGREDIENTS

*1 packet Micro Chicken Soup*
*1 packet Micro Pea Soup*
*½ medium onion, diced small*
*2 stalks celery, diced small*
*1 lb. asparagus, diced small*
*1 cup skim milk*
*Mrs. Dash "Onions & Herbs"*

PROCEDURE

Saute onion and celery in non-stick pan until soft. Place in pot with 2 cups water and asparagus. Cook uncovered for approximately 15 minutes, or until asparagus is very soft. Add skim milk and heat until warm. Mix in Micro Soups, stir well, and serve hot. (Serves 2)

PER SERVING:

| | |
|---|---|
| Calories - 155 | Fat - 2 gm |
| Protein - 15.6 gm | % of fat - 12% |
| Carbohydrate - 25 gm | Sodium - 423 mg |

## ■ A CASE STUDY

### SYLVIA RAMSEY: A DRESS FOR SUCCESS

Sylvia Ramsey's doctor started her on The Micro Diet program after telling her she was a "walking time bomb." Sylvia, age forty-one, weighed 268 pounds and her cholesterol level, she says, was sky-high.

"I felt like I had one foot in the grave and was doomed to be heavy the rest of my life. I was weighed down by personal problems and I ate my misery away. I was a foodaholic. I was a constant all-day eater. I would go for fast foods because they were fast and easy and I got into the bad habit of frying everything. When I felt tired the first thing I would grab for a quick pick-me-up would be a candy bar or ice cream. I never found time to put together a balanced meal. I suspect I was hungry all the time because I just wasn't getting any real nutrition, so my body wasn't satisfied."

A mother of five, Sylvia, of Provo, Utah, says that she had been heavy most of her life and had tried countless diets, but was always hungry, and moody, and thinking of what to fix for her next meal. "I got to the point where I believed there really wasn't a solution." But, under doctor's orders she determined to try one more diet, The Micro Diet. To her astonishment, she enjoyed the taste and didn't feel hungry. The variety of meals, she says, meant that she was never bored and, in the first month, she dropped twenty pounds.

"I felt like a light bulb had been turned on inside my head and I started smiling again. My face started to look alive. I couldn't believe this was a diet. I felt too good. I didn't feel deprived. I had so much energy that I was motivated to stick with it. The fact that the meals were already prepared made it so much easier for me. It took my mind off of having to fix meals."

To set herself a serious goal, Sylvia deliberately bought a beautiful pink dress that was a size nine—several sizes too small for her. "I left it in plain view hanging out over my closet. Whenever I needed a motivational boost, I would go and look at it and say to myself 'I'm going to get in this dress.' You can't imagine how excited I was when that finally happened and I wore it to a special occasion."

Getting into that dress meant that Sylvia had lost a total of 125 pounds. After maintaining that weight loss for over a year, she says,

"I'm free from my weight problem. I could shout with joy, 'The Micro Diet works!' I feel wonderful. I feel like I've got a second chance at life. I've pulled out of my depression. My self-esteem is back. I sleep better and wake up in the mornings full of energy. This morning I got up around 5:00 A.M., weeded the yard, and pulled some raspberries. I then took my mother shopping, and later came home and took another friend shopping. After that, I spent two hours perming my daughter's hair. Tonight I'm going to a meeting and will go to bed about 11:00 P.M. And this is a typical day for me."

To maintain her new figure, Sylvia continues to enjoy two Micro Diet meals a day, as well as using Micro meals when preparing other dishes. "In my home, The Micro Diet is a common household item on the shelf. I use this food in other meals that I prepare for the family to give extra nutrition to their diet as well as mine. For instance, I pour the soup mixes into stews or stove-top dressing mixes. I add the chicken soup when I roast chicken. When I make ice-cream malts for the kids, I put a few packets of the shake mixes into each batch. The Micro Diet is something that you just have to have in the pantry like flour and seasonings. I keep a jar of Micro Diet shake mix on the counter next to the jars of flour and sugar, so the kids can scoop it into their drinks for extra energy and nutrition."

Adds Sylvia, "It's amazing how differently I look at food now. I still want food that is quick and easy, and that is the main reason why The Micro Diet works so well for me. There are too many times when I'm running out the door and I only have time to grab something quick. I now reach for a Micro bar instead of a candy bar. I've replaced some old bad habits with new, more positive ones. I'm not hungry all the time. My craving for sweets and unhealthy eating has disappeared.

"The old Sylvia is past history and the Sylvia I always wanted to be is now a reality. My husband can put both arms around me with room to spare, and I'm looking and feeling like the girl he married."

# 9

# BETTER THAN MOTHER USED TO MAKE

"IF YOU WANT YOUR FAMILY to eat right," says Susan Meyerott, M.S., creator of *Choices*—The Micro Diet's lifestyle enhancement program, "you've got to make that healthy food look and taste like the foods they like. When you serve your family a healthy meal and they ask for 'more' instead of asking 'what's this?' you know you've created the perfect meal."

Susan, a physiologist who takes a very personal, practical approach to adjusting habits, spent ten years teaching at the University of California in Los Angeles and at the Center for Health Enhancement Education and Research at UCLA. She figures if she can get herself and her family to eat better, she can get other people to do the same.

"When I was asked to develop *Choices*, I had just delivered my second child, and was fatter and more out of shape than I had ever been. After being sick for nine months and gaining weight 'just fine,' I was looking forward to eating and being fat for awhile. When I was asked to develop a weight management program, I thought it was one of God's little jokes. I decided to accept the challenge—and work on my own weight at the same time."

Susan spent the next year developing *Choices*, experimenting with Micro meals, and losing thirty-five pounds in the process. Two years later she's kept the weight off.

"I'm a traditional health professional, who was taught that the term 'convenience food' automatically meant unhealthy. So

I almost turned my nose up at the thought of incorporating 'pre-packaged' meals in my diet. But faced with taking a significant amount of weight off myself—one more time—I was forced to look at The Micro Diet, not just through the eyes of the know-it-all expert, but also through the eyes of a dieter, and the eyes of a mother.

"The expert in me looked for sound nutrition; the dieter looked for a simple, but flexible approach; and the mother looked for nutritious food my children (and husband) would actually eat. What I discovered were foods that provided excellent nutrition in ten minutes or less, that were easy to incorporate into hundreds of different meals the entire family would eat."

In the *Choices* program, Susan shows people how to enhance their life, attitude, and nutrition by making small adjustments rather than major changes. In this section, she shows us just how easy it is to make small changes in traditional recipes to enhance family meals.

"It's the small changes over a lifetime that add up," says Susan. "You don't have to give up eating your favorite foods to be healthier. Be willing to experiment with Micro meals to find ways to fix your favorite recipes so they provide more nutrition and less fat."

Compare the nutritional profiles of the traditional recipes with the enhanced ones below. Then experiment with the enhanced versions, and discover for yourself just how good enhanced meals can taste.

## SUNDAY MORNING BRUNCH MENU

*(Breakfast for Four)*

Banana–Blueberry Muesli Muffins
Orange Juice
Papaya with Vanilla Yogurt, topped with Strawberry
Coffee (adults)
Nonfat Milk (kids)

*Per Person Serving*

3 Banana–Blueberry Muesli Muffins
½ cup orange juice
½ papaya with ¼ cup vanilla yogurt topped with 1 large strawberry
coffee (adults)
1 glass nonfat milk (kids)

| | WITHOUT MILK | WITH MILK |
|---|---|---|
| Calories: | 433 | 519 |
| Protein: | 19 grams | 27 grams |
| Fat: | 8 grams (16%) | 8 grams (14%) |
| Fiber: | 5.4 grams | 5.4 grams |
| Sodium: | 531 mgs | 657 mgs |

# BLUEBERRY MUFFINS

**Traditional**
**Bisquick Blueberry Muffins**

*1 large egg*
*2 cups Bisquick*
*⅓ cup sugar*
*⅔ cup 1% milk*
*2 tablespoons vegetable oil*
*¾ cup unsweetened frozen blueberries*

**Enhanced**
**Banana-Blueberry Muesli Muffins**

*1 large egg*
*½ cup Bisquick*
*2 ripe bananas, sliced*
*½ cup 1% milk*
*½ cup unsweetened frozen blueberries*
*2 packets Micro Muesli*
*1 teaspoon cinnamon*

Preheat oven to 375 degrees. Beat egg slightly in large mixing bowl; stir in remaining ingredients except blueberries until just moistened. Fold in blueberries. Spray muffin pan with non-stick spray or use paper cups to line. Bake 18–20 minutes. Both provide 4 servings or 24 mini-muffins.

PER RECIPE
Calories: 1639
Protein: 28 grams
Fat: 67 grams (36%)
Fiber: 1.7 grams
Sodium: 3049 mg

PER 3 MUFFIN SERVING
Calories: 411
Protein: 7 grams
Fat: 17 grams (36%)
Fiber: less than 1 gram
Sodium: 735 mg

PER RECIPE
Calories: 1141
Protein: 51 grams
Fat: 24 grams (18%)
Fiber: 19 grams
Sodium: 1828 mg

PER 3 MUFFIN SERVING
Calories: 285
Protein: 13 grams
Fat: 6 grams (18%)
Fiber: 4.7 grams
Sodium: 456 mg

## SUNDAY MORNING BRUNCH MENU

Champagne and Pancakes

Fruit and Muesli Pancakes topped with Fresh Strawberries
and Low-fat Lemon or Strawberry Yogurt
Champagne
Coffee

*Per Person*
3 fruit & Muesli pancakes
¼ cup low-fat lemon or strawberry yogurt
¼ cup sliced fresh strawberries
1 glass champagne

| | WITH CHAMPAGNE | WITHOUT CHAMPAGNE |
|---|---|---|
| Calories: | 425 | 341 |
| Protein: | 15 grams | 15 grams |
| Fat: | 6 grams (13%) | 6 grams (16%) |
| Fiber: | 5 grams | 5 grams |
| Sodium: | 492 mg | 492 mg |

# PANCAKES

**Traditional Bisquick Pancakes**

*2 cups Bisquick*
*2 eggs*
*1 cup 1% milk*

**Enhanced Fruit & Muesli Pancakes**

*½ cup Bisquick*
*2 packets Micro Muesli*
*1 egg*
*½ cup nonfat milk*
*¾ cup water*
*1 ripe banana, sliced*
*1 apple, diced with skin*
*¼ cup unsweetened frozen blueberries*
*1 teaspoon cinnamon*

Beat all ingredients except fruit until well blended. Add cut up fruit and mix. Cook on medium heat. Pour onto hot pan sprayed with non-stick spray. Cook on medium heat until edges are dry. Turn; cook until golden.

Both recipes provide 4 servings or 12 pancakes per recipe (or 24 mini-pancakes)

PER TRADITIONAL RECIPE
Calories: 1212
Protein: 37 grams
Fat: 45 grams (33%)
Fiber: 0
Sodium: 3049 mg

PER 3 PANCAKE SERVING
Calories: 303
Protein: 10 grams
Fat: 11 grams (33%)
Fiber: 0
Sodium: 762 mg

PER ENHANCED RECIPE
Calories: 1090
Protein: 50 grams
Fat: 23 grams (18%)
Fiber: 19 grams
Sodium: 1834 mg

PER 3 PANCAKE SERVING
Calories: 274
Protein: 12.5 grams
Fat: 6 grams (18%)
Fiber: 5 grams
Sodium: 459 mg

## SATURDAY MORNING BREAKFAST

*(For Four)*

Apple Cinnamon Waffles Topped with Fresh Fruit
Orange Juice
Coffee

PER PERSON

Two 3″ x 3″ apple-cinnamon waffles
1 cup mixed fruit topping
½ cup orange juice
coffee

NUTRITIONAL INFORMATION PER SERVING

Calories: 401
Protein: 15 grams
Fat: 6 grams (14%)
Fiber: 7 grams
Sodium: 461 mg

# WAFFLES

**Traditional Waffles**

*2 cups Bisquick*
*2 eggs*
*1 cup 1% milk*

**Enhanced Cinnamon-Apple Muesli Waffles**

*½ cup Bisquick*
*2 packets Micro Muesli*
*1 egg*
*½ cup nonfat milk*
*¾ cup water*
*1 ripe banana, sliced*
*1 apple, diced with skin*
*1½ teaspoon cinnamon*

Preheat waffle iron. Beat egg in large mixing bowl; stir in remaining ingredients. Spray waffle iron with non-stick spray. Pour batter onto center of hot waffle iron. Bake until steaming stops. Makes two nine-inch waffles, or eight three-inch waffles.

Both recipes make four servings of two-to-three, three-inch waffles.

*Nutritional Information for Waffles*

PER TRADITIONAL RECIPE
Calories: 1212
Protein: 37 grams
Fat: 47 grams (33%)
Fiber: 0
Sodium: 3049 mg

PER SERVING
Calories: 303
Protein: 9 grams
Fat: 11 grams (33%)
Fiber: 0
Sodium: 762 mg

PER ENHANCED RECIPE
Calories: 1073
Protein: 50 grams
Fat: 22 grams (18%)
Fiber: 18 grams
Sodium: 1834 mg

PER SERVING
Calories: 268
Protein: 13 grams
Fat: 6 grams (18%)
Fiber: 5 grams
Sodium: 459 mg

# PANCAKE AND WAFFLE TOPPINGS

**Traditional**
**Syrup & Butter Topping**

*2 cups pancake syrup*
*12 tablespoons butter*

*Butter, then pour!*

**Enhanced**
**Fresh Fruit Topping**

*1 banana, sliced*
*1 cup fresh sliced strawberries*
*1 cup unsweetened frozen raspberries*
*1 cup unsweetened frozen blackberries*

*Mix cut up fruit together. Serve over waffles or pancakes.*

*Both recipes make four servings*

*Nutritional Information for Waffles with Toppings*

PER TRADITIONAL RECIPE
Calories: 4332
Protein: 38 grams
Fat: 181 grams (38%)
Fiber: 0
Sodium: 5561 mg

PER SERVING
Calories: 1083
Protein: 9 grams
Fat: 45 grams (38%)
Fiber: 0
Sodium: 1390 mg

PER ENHANCED RECIPE
Calories: 1381
Protein: 55 grams
Fat: 25 grams (16%)
Fiber: 28 grams
Sodium: 1839 mg

PER SERVING
Calories: 345
Protein: 14 grams
Fat: 6 grams (16%)
Fiber: 7 grams
Sodium: 460 mg

# TOSTADA

**Traditional Tostada**

*2 corn tortilla*
*1 cup shredded lettuce*
*1 green onion, diced*
*1 ripe tomato, diced*
*1 cup refried beans*
*½ cup cheddar cheese*
*2 tablespoons sour half and half cream*
*¼ cup oil & vinegar dressing*
*¼ cup salsa*

**Enhanced Chili Tostada**

*2 corn tortilla*
*1 cup shredded lettuce*
*1 green onion, diced*
*1 ripe tomato, diced*
*1 packet Micro Chili, prepared*
*½ cup salsa*
*2 tablespoons sour half & half cream*

Warm up refried beans on the stove or in the microwave (or prepare the Micro Chili by adding one cup boiled water to the Micro Chili, then letting it stand in a covered bowl for 10 minutes). Cut up lettuce, onion, tomato, (cheese), and place them in serving bowls. Crisp tortilla in a skillet sprayed with non-stick spray, cooking over medium-high heat for 30 seconds each side, or warm up in the oven or microwave. Place tortilla on plate and layer with beans or chili, then rest of ingredients, and choice of dressing. Top with sour cream.

Serves One*

*Yes, it could serve two but what are your real portions?

*Nutritional Information for Tostada*

PER TRADITIONAL RECIPE
Calories: 1032
Fat: 63 grams (52%)
Fiber: 9.7 grams
Sodium: 1999 mg

PER ENHANCED RECIPE
Calories: 458
Fat: 9.5 grams (17%)
Fiber: 5.6 grams
Sodium: 1177 mg

# CHILI

**Traditional Chili Con Carne With Tomatoes**

*½ lb. ground beef*
*1 medium onion, chopped*
*½ cup chopped green pepper*
*1 ripe tomato, chopped*
*1 small can tomato sauce*
*1 teaspoon chili powder*
*½ teaspoon salt*
*dash cayenne red pepper*

*½ (15½ oz.) can kidney beans*
*2 cups water*

**Enhanced Micro Chili Con Carne and Tomatoes**

*¼ lb. extra lean ground beef*
*½ medium onion, chopped*
*½ cup choped green pepper*
*1 ripe tomato, chopped*
*½ teaspoon chili powder*
*a dash cayenne red pepper*
*¼ teaspoon salt*

*2 packets Micro Chili*

Cook and stir ground beef, onion, and green pepper in skillet until meat is brown and onion tender. For Micro Chili: While beef mixture cooking, heat two cups water, stir into Micro Chili, and let stand in a covered bowl for ten minutes. Stir in remaining ingredients to beef mixture, add to the Micro Chili. Serves two. For traditional recipe: Stir in remaining ingredients, except kidney beans, and bring to a boil, then reduce heat; and simmer uncovered forty-five minutes, stirring occasionally. Stir in beans; heat. Serves two.

*Nutritional Information for Chili*

PER TRADITIONAL RECIPE
Calories: 855
Fat: 44 grams (46%)
Fiber: 5 grams
Sodium: 2438 mg

PER SERVING:
Calories: 427
Fat: 22 grams (46%)
Fiber: 2.5 grams
Sodium: 1219 mg

PER ENHANCED RECIPE
Calories: 811
Fat: 23 grams (25%)
Fiber: 11 grams
Sodium: 1848 mg

PER SERVING
Calories: 405
Fat: 12 grams (27%)
Fiber: 5 grams
Sodium: 924 mg

# PESTO FOR TWO

**Traditional**
**Fettucini Noodles**
**with Pesto Sauce**

*2 cups cooked fettucini noodles*
*1 cup fresh/frozen peas*
*½ cup fresh mushrooms, chopped*
*2 tablespoons oil*
*½ cup grated Parmesan cheese*
*2 tablespoons chopped fresh basil*
*½ cup walnuts*
*1 garlic clove*
*2 teaspoons salt*

**Enhanced**
**Tetrazzini with**
**Pesto Sauce**

*2 Micro Chicken Tetrazzini packets, prepared as directed*
*½ cup fresh/frozen peas*
*½ cup fresh mushrooms, chopped*
*2 tablespoons grated Parmesan cheese*
*2 tablespoons chopped fresh basil*
*2 tablespoons walnuts*
*1 garlic clove*
*1 teaspoon salt*

Cook noodles in boiling water; drain (or add boiling water to tetrazzini and let stand in covered bowl). Grind (oil), Parmesan cheese, basil, walnuts, garlic, and salt in blender until coarsely ground. Add to cooked noodles and lightly toss. Add chopped mushrooms and frozen peas (uncooked). Serves two.

*Nutritional Information for Traditional and Enchanced Recipe*

PER TRADITIONAL RECIPE
Calories: 1358
Fat: 78 grams (51%)
Fiber: 8 grams
Sodium: 5578 mg

PER SERVING
Calories: 679
Fat: 39 grams (51%)
Fiber: 4 grams
Sodium: 2789 mg

PER ENHANCED RECIPE
Calories: 760
Fat: 16 grams (18%)
Fiber: 4 grams
Sodium: 4118 mg

PER SERVING
Calories: 380
Fat: 8 grams (18%)
Fiber: 2 grams
Sodium: 2059 mg

# FRUIT SALAD

**Traditional**
**Fruit Salad with Fluffy Fruit Dressing**

*½ cup watermelon*
*1 banana*
*1 peach*
*½ cup strawberries*
*1 kiwi fruit*
*½ cup cantaloupe*
*½ cup marshmallows*
*1 tablespoon orange juice*
*2½ tablespoons salad dressing*
*¼ teaspoon vanilla extract*

**Enhanced**
**Fruit Lover's Delight**

*½ cup watermelon*
*1 banana*
*1 peach*
*½ cup strawberries*
*1 kiwi fruit*
*½ cup cantaloupe*
*¼ cup water*
*1 packet Micro Strawberry Drink*
*1 tablespoon orange juice*

Cut up fruit into large bowl. Mix other ingredients together in a blender, pour over fruit; mix and chill. Serves one.

*Nutritional Information for Fruit Salad with Dressing*

PER TRADITIONAL RECIPE
Calories: 813
Fat: 22 grams (23%)
Fiber: 3 grams
Sodium: 59 mg

PER ENHANCED RECIPE
Calories: 481
Fat: 4 grams (7%)
Fiber: 3 grams
Sodium: 516 mg

Note: This is a complete meal for one person. The Micro strawberry dressing provides 35% of your daily requirements for all vitamins, minerals, trace elements, and protein.

*Recipe courtesy Charlie Brown, Arizona*

## PUDDING (DESSERT)

**Traditional**
**Rice Pudding**

*1 cup cooked brown rice*
*dash salt*
*½ cup sugar*
*1 tablespoon cornstarch*
*2 large eggs*
*2½ cups milk (2%)*
*1 tablespoon lemon juice*
*½ cup raisins*
*¼ cup sugar*

**Enhanced**
**Creamy Rice and Muesli Pudding**

*⅔ cup cooked brown rice*
*dash salt*
*2 tablespoons sugar*
*1 tablespoon cornstarch*
*1 large egg*
*1 cup nonfat milk*
*¼ cup lemon juice*
*1 tablespoon lemon peel*
*1 packet Micro Muesli*
*1 cup water*
*1 teaspoon cinnamon*
*2 tablespoons sugar*

Blend sugar, cornstarch, and salt in top of double boiler. Separate egg(s); beat egg yolk slightly, and put egg white aside. Add egg yolk and milk/water to sugar/cornstarch; beat. Stir in rice (muesli), lemon juice, lemon peel, cinnamon, and raisins. Place over bottom of double boiler filled with water. Cook for twenty minutes at medium-high heat, stirring occasionally, or until pudding is creamy and most of liquid is absorbed. Remove from stove and place in glass baking dish sprayed with a non-stick spray. Preheat oven to 400 degrees. Beat egg whites until foamy. Beat in two tablespoons (or ¼ cup) sugar, adding one tablespoon at a time; continue beating until stiff and glossy. Spread on pudding. Bake 8–10 minutes or until meringue is golden brown. Serve warm. Just before serving sprinkle pudding with cinnamon. Serves four.

*Nutritional Information for Traditional and Enchanced Pudding*

PER TRADITIONAL PUDDING RECIPE
Calories: 1460
Fat: 24 grams (14%)
Fiber: 1.6 grams
Sodium: 500 mg

PER SERVING
Calories: 365
Fat: 6 grams (14%)
Fiber: .4 grams
Sodium: 125 mg

PER ENHANCED PUDDING RECIPE
Calories: 907
Fat: 11 grams (10%)
Fiber: 9.5 grams
Sodium: 708 mg

PER SERVING
Calories: 227
Fat: 6 grams (10%)
Fiber: 2.4 grams
Sodium: 177 mg

## *SAMPLE MICRO MEAL 1,000–1,200 CALORIE MENU*

## *WEEK 1*

| MON | TUES | WED | THUR | FRI | SAT | SUN |
|---|---|---|---|---|---|---|
| | | | ***BREAKFAST*** | | | |
| Muesli with Rice | Chocolate Drink | Peanut Bar | Strawberry Drink | Banana Blueberry Muesli Muffins (3) | Fruit & Muesli Pancakes w/fruit | Cinnamon-Apple Muesli Waffles w/fruit |
| | | | ***LUNCH*** | | | |
| Crunchy Peanut Bar | Tomato Soup | Vanilla Drink | Banana Blueberry Muesli Muffins (3) | Pea Soup | Chicken Soup | Chocolate Drink |
| | | | ***DINNER*** | | | |
| Chili | Manhattan Clam Chowder | Cream of Asparagus Soup | Spanish Rice | Chicken Tetrazzini | Spicy Shrimp Roll-ups | Tomato Soup |
| | | | ***SNACK*** | | | |
| Chicken Soup | | | Banana Blueberry Muesli Muffins (3) | Banana Blueberry Mueseli Muffins (3) | | |

Recipes for meals listed in these weekly menu plans can be found in chapters 8 and 9.

## *DAILY TOTALS*

| MON | TUES | WED | THUR | FRI | SAT | SUN |
|---|---|---|---|---|---|---|
| ***CALORIES*** | | | | | | |
| 966 cal | 851 cal | 1091 cal | 1037 cal | 1060 cal | 985 cal | 794 cal |
| ***PROTEIN (GRAMS)*** | | | | | | |
| 73 gms | 69 gms | 99 gms | 64 gms | 63 gms | 79 gms | 56 gms |
| ***FAT (GRAMS)*** | | | | | | |
| 16 gms | 9 gms | 16 gms | 15 gms | 17 gms | 14 gms | 12 gms |
| ***FAT (PERCENT)*** | | | | | | |
| 14% | 10% | 13% | 13% | 15% | 13% | 13% |
| ***FIBER (GRAMS)*** | | | | | | |
| 16 gms | 4 gms | 13 gms | 11 gms | 10 gms | 9 gms | 8 gms |
| ***SODIUM (MILLIGRAMS)*** | | | | | | |
| 2077 mg | 2042 mg | 2693 mg | 2165 mg | 2455 mg | 1935 mg | 1659 mg |

## *SAMPLE MICRO MEAL 1,000–1,200 CALORIE MENU*

## *WEEK 2*

| MON | TUES | WED | THUR | FRI | SAT | SUN |
|---|---|---|---|---|---|---|
| | | | ***BREAKFAST*** | | | |
| Muesli Cereal | Hot Chocolate Drink | Peanut Bar | Hot Strawberry Drink | Muesli Bar | Hot Chocolate Drink | Crunchy Peanut Bar |
| | | | ***LUNCH*** | | | |
| Peanut Bar | Tomato Soup | Strawberry Smoothie | Yogurt-Orange Bar | Pea Soup | Chili | Chicken Soup |
| | | | ***DINNER*** | | | |
| Chili Tostada | Spanish Rice & Couscous (½ recipe) | Fruit Lovers Delight | Stuffed Manicotti | Gazpacho (½ recipe) | Chicken Newburg | Spaghetti Squash Alfredo |

## *DAILY TOTALS*

| MON | TUES | WED | THUR | FRI | SAT | SUN |
|---|---|---|---|---|---|---|
| | | | ***CALORIES*** | | | |
| 978 cal | 937 cal | 1003 cal | 1061 cal | 993 cal | 931 cal | 886 cal |
| | | | ***PROTEIN (GRAMS)*** | | | |
| 56 gms | 67 gms | 64 gms | 77 gms | 62 gms | 80 gms | 61 gms |
| | | | ***FAT (GRAMS)*** | | | |
| 20 gms | 9 gms | 12 gms | 28 gms | 14 gms | 8 gms | 17 gms |
| | | | ***FAT (PERCENT)*** | | | |
| 17% | 8% | 10% | 23% | 12% | 8% | 16% |
| | | | ***FIBER (GRAMS)*** | | | |
| 22 gms | 4 gms | 12 gms | 5 gms | 12 gms | 5 gms | 6 gms |
| | | | ***SODIUM (MILLIGRAMS)*** | | | |
| 2177 mg | 2026 mg | 1518 mg | 1381 mg | 2033 mg | 2046 mg | 1897 mg |

## ■ A CASE STUDY

### BRYCE AND BONNIE BLEDSOE: D-DAY WAS A GOOD DAY

Husband and wife Bryce and Bonnie Bledsoe of Bakersfield, California, decided to diet together and, after receiving The Micro Diet on a Tuesday, did what so many would-be dieters do: They procrastinated. They decided that the following Monday would be "D" for Diet day. That gave them almost a whole week to prepare for their diet—by hitting every "all you can eat" restaurant in town.

Says Bryce, "You know how it is when you go on a diet. You know that you are going to starve yourself, so you want to make sure you get as much food as you can into your system before you start."

D-Day arrived and the Bledsoes, both age sixty, each had a shake for breakfast, a bar for lunch, and the Micro Chili for dinner, seemingly very little food by their normal eating pattern. Then they sat down in their easy chairs to watch television. As the evening went by they kept looking at each other and were astonished to find they didn't feel the need for an evening snack. The next day was a repeat performance. "We just weren't hungry. We felt great. Our minds told us that we should have more to eat, but our bodies were satisfied," says Bryce. Says Bonnie, "That entire first evening neither one of us got up to get something to eat. The following morning I said to Bryce, 'I never want to be without this.' I had energy. I wasn't dragging myself out of bed."

Bryce always had a weight problem. He weighed 150 pounds when he was ten years old. "I was raised on the farm so, at that age, I was doing a man's work for fifty cents a day and my lunch. And they fed you a man's portion." Bryce was 249 pounds when he graduated from high school and eventually reached 385 pounds. "I was so large I could barely walk half a block. It got to the point that I couldn't bend over to tie my own shoelaces." After losing 108 pounds (with another forty-five to go), he says, "We don't just sit at home watching TV, playing cards, and eating anymore. We have choices in our lives. We do a lot of walking and I can tie my own shoelaces.

"We no longer have the desire for the kinds of food that we gained our weight with. We have found that if we eat from salad bars we feel fine. If we eat red meats we feel sluggish. This is the first time I've ever been able to watch the food commercials on TV and not head for the kitchen to get something to eat. Bonnie and I both had a big problem with overeating. We can't believe that we have that under control. When we go out now, we eat sensibly instead of eating until we can't hold any more. We know that with The Micro Diet we won't regain our weight."

When Bryce started The Micro Diet, he was visiting his doctor every two weeks to have his blood pressure checked. After losing ninety-five pounds in seventeen weeks, he discovered that it had dropped from 200/110 to 168/90. Bonnie lost seventy-five pounds in the same time and her cholesterol dropped frm 219 to 192, and triglycerides from 395 to 241. The couple used The Micro Diet as their sole source of nutrition for the first two weeks, and then ate out one night a week, selecting baked or broiled fish and baked potato, and salad. They ordered dressing on the side and contented themselves with just dipping their forks into it. After six weeks, they began eating out twice a week.

Five-foot, two-inch Bonnie, who weighed 317 pounds, has now lost a total of eighty-seven pounds and wants to lose another sixty pounds. She says, "When Bryce and I first met one another we found we had so much in common—especially our love of eating and in particular the 'eat all you want' places. We wanted all of our money's worth and we were never satisfied. We could stuff ourselves to the point where we were miserable. You would be amazed at the amount of food we could eat.

"When I was a child everything centered around food. You were rewarded with food. 'Be a good girl, Bonnie Jean, and I'll give you a cookie when you get home.' Family get-togethers were always major eating occasions, so I learned that food and companionship go hand-in-hand. The Micro Diet has taught us that we can still enjoy company and eat good food, and not suffer."

Best of all, says Bonnie, is the satisfaction of going out for an occasional meal without the dinner triggering a binge-eating attack. "Knowing that I can have that meal, not feel guilty about it, and not blow the entire diet has really kept me going. I have lost weight on so many diets before, but if I went off the diet just for one meal I found it almost impossible to get back on the diet. But this is more than a diet. It has changed our lives completely. It is something we are going to live with for the rest of our lives, not because we have to but because we want to."

# 10

# THE HELPING HAND

EVERYBODY NEEDS SOMEBODY. And with The Micro Diet, when you lose weight, you do so with the friendly support and encouragement of an Independent Micro Diet distributor, called an "Advisor," because so much of what he or she does goes beyond just supplying the diet to you. This personal Advisor is assigned to you as soon as you begin the program; someone, most probably, who has also fought the weight-loss battle and can counsel you by providing the benefit of his or her own personal experience—free of charge.

Some weight-control programs insist that you visit a storefront center to attend fixed appointments. Undoubtedly, that works for some dieters. My observation is that for most people the Advisor system works better by providing more personalized support whenever the dieter wants it and without the cost of attending a "clinic," which, as one critic pointed out, can be staffed by "young women who are size ten and chide you like a child for gaining a pound."

This individualized service is the one I'm familiar with, and have observed its benefits firsthand. Let me describe it for you. The Advisor might work with you by phone, visit you in the privacy of your home, or even open up his or her own home to work with you in a comfortable, nonintimidating environment. Many Advisors and dieters also find it extremely beneficial to get together for group sessions either in dieters' homes, hotels, or other meeting places.

Certainly, you can also "go it alone" and not take advantage of an Advisor's experience. It's your choice. But many studies have shown that your prospects of success are greatly improved if you have the benefit of a support system.

There is now an army of thousands of Micro Diet Advisors throughout the world sharing with dieters the ups and downs of their own struggle and keeping them supplied with Micro meals. They are able to say "I've tried it, and it works," and they are able to answer your basic questions. Some of them are trained health professionals; most are not. Their role is to be "helping hands" or friends, not experts, even if they are health professionals. If you need medical advice you should see your personal physician or dietitian.

The Advisor has the time to spend with you in whatever way you choose, time that the busy doctor or dietitian does not have—yet another example of the flexibility of the program.

## *TOO GOOD TO BE TRUE*

In many parts of the country, meetings are held to discuss how to use the diet, and dieters share their experiences. The spirit of togetherness generated at such meetings is often the decisive factor influencing dieters to take the first vital step toward achieving their goal.

I vividly remember one meeting held in a small church hall in a suburb of Birmingham, England. It was the middle of winter and only twenty people had turned out. There were a handful of Advisors, some dieters who had begun to lose weight, and others who were hearing about the program for the first time. We discussed how the diet had been devised and developed. We talked about the fact that some people do not have a satisfactory weight loss on 1,500 calories a day, and I explained that using The Micro Diet as one's sole source of nutrition offered real hope for such people. I went on to relate some of the success stories of our dieters.

There was one very large lady listening most attentively, frequently nodding her head in agreement with the points I was making. She seemed to have no doubts about the logic. She had come to the meeting, however, with a thin friend, presumably for moral support. At the end of the presentation, after I had thanked everyone for attending, the thin friend exclaimed loudly so that the whole room could hear, "Bah! Sounds too good to be true!"

Before I had a chance to respond, a woman sitting behind them tapped the thin one on the shoulder and said, to my delight, "That's exactly what I said two months and thirty pounds ago." The cloud of doubt which had passed over the face of the large lady disappeared instantly.

It was not the first nor the last time I have heard such skepticism. I fully understand the skepticism, as I was once a skeptic myself, and it is highly likely that they have already tried many different ways of losing weight—and failed. They have already experienced the misery of slow dispiriting weight loss, of giving up in failure or, if they were among the few to reach goal weight, found that the fat came piling back on. To be told that average weight losses of fourteen pounds a month can be achieved obtaining complete nutrition in a mere 800 calories, while feeling well and full of energy, certainly does sound too good to be true.

Joan Shepler, of Austell, Georgia, says that the "ultimate realization" of just how much The Micro Diet meant to her came when she was invited to be the star guest at a weekly meeting. Husband Bill went along and asked for permission to introduce her. Then, at the appropriate moment, he surprised her by lugging a pair of forty-pound dumbbells to the front of the crowd, and, after letting them crash to the floor, announced that was how much she had lost.

Says forty-eight-year-old Joan, "The audience was aghast and it made me suddenly realize the extra burden that had been on my heart." Joan, who went on to get rid of ninety-five pounds, and has kept it off more than a year, adds, "The whole experience has been so exhilarating that I'm almost at a loss for words. My exercise program has also paid off. My legs are no longer flabby and my insect-like protruding abdomen is gone. I'm actually firm."

Best of all, says Joan, she knows just how much her new figure means to her husband, a prominent health and fitness expert. "When I was overweight, it was undoubtedly a source of embarrassment for him. I had unwittingly been placing him in the category of the shoemaker whose kids are barefoot. Now I hear him joking to our friends that he feels guilty, like he is having an affair, because of the strange woman in bed with him at night."

Attendance at meetings is purely on a voluntary basis. Perhaps instead, you would prefer your Advisor to visit you in your home for a small group meeting or a personal chat; or perhaps you would like to keep in contact by telephone. Advisors are used to fielding phone calls at home. If it helps to keep you on a continuing weight-loss pattern, they feel it is time well spent. Your Advisor will be happy to help you, whichever way you see fit. The praise we have received for the overall quality of the Advisor network is most encouraging.

Thirty-one-year-old Connie Reeder, who lost 107 pounds in a year, says she couldn't have done it without the helping hand of her Micro Diet Advisor, Debbie Heath. "She's always been there for me. She's become a second mother," says Connie. "Debbie has really taken a personal interest in me and makes sure that my head is on straight. I know that she must have a whole directory of people that she keeps in contact with, but she makes me feel like I'm the only one. I like the fact that she doesn't compare her dieters. She has taught me that everyone loses weight differently."

Particularly during the weight-loss phase, Debbie gave her a wealth of practical advice, says Connie, including how to alternate the various Micro Diet plans so she never ran the risk of becoming bored with her diet. "She gave me lots of direction and lots of friendly encouragement. She taught me all the variations I could make for 300 calories, because I was so afraid of blowing it. She would have me write down everything that I ate and every week would go over it with me so I could plan better for the next week."

Through Debbie, Connie met other Advisors in the Brantford, Ontario, area. "They are a very big part of my life. They help you along with the dieting and reassure you if you regain a few pounds and need to get back on track. Their encouragement and help goes hand-in-hand with the dieting."

Connie had been overweight since her teens thanks to a heavy junk food diet of hamburgers, pizza, cookies, chips, popcorn, and soda. When she noticed friends losing weight with The Micro Diet, she decided to try it for herself. "It was hard at first but it soon became a fun routine, especially when I saw the weight coming off and could fit into smaller size clothing again. I looked good and I felt good. It was the first diet I have ever been able to stick to."

Connie's advice to new dieters: Don't give up. "If someone feels that they have blown it one day, so what? One day is nothing overall. When that happened to me, Debbie would tell me, 'That day is gone, so get back on track and don't be hard on yourself. It's only one day. Just pick up where you left off.' And that's exactly what I would say to anyone starting The Micro Diet."

Connie, a preschool teacher, says, "I love that I can now cross my legs and get down to the kids' level. Before losing the weight I was not able to get down on the floor. I'm proud of the way I look. I like to be able to tuck my shirt in and put a belt around my waist, instead of wearing smock-type clothing."

Connie is not alone in recognizing the unusual support network. I've even heard about one extremely overweight man who was agoraphobic and would not venture outside his front door. He had not been able to get any help until his Micro Diet Advisor visited him in the privacy of his own home. Disabled people have been aided in the same way. The personal contact is an integral part of the system. You, the dieter, have the example of the Advisor as a visible sign that the diet plan works. Quite often, the Advisor may still be on the weight-loss path himself or herself, treading step-by-step with you.

The Advisor provides you with the latest Micro Diet information, whether it's nutritional guidelines, recipes, menu-planning, or even new Micro meals. The Advisor can also introduce you to *Choices*, our lifestyle modification program. Most of all, the Advisor is simply someone to provide the encouragement and motivation for you to triumph once and for all over your weight problem.

In Beth Cullop's case, the encouragement arrived with a surprise UPS delivery, a Micro Diet variety pack from her sister, with a note simply saying, "Don't ask any questions. Just do it." She did. And lost twenty pounds in the first two and a half weeks, sixty pounds in two and a half months, and has now gotten rid of a total of 120 pounds from a top weight of 258. She's also slipping into a size eight instead of a tight twenty-two. And she's another long-term loser, having maintained her ideal weight for over a year.

Says thirty-six-year-old Beth, of Blaine, Washington, "If it had not been for my sister becoming an Advisor and loving me enough and caring enough about my health, I would never have tried it. She was with me all the way. Having her to talk to whenever

I needed made all the difference. I was always a late-night muncher. Then my sister suggested that I eat my final Micro meal just before bed. So each night at bedtime I ate a bar, gradually eating less and less of a bar until my habit was broken."

Beverly Smith of Hurst, Texas, turned losing weight into a family affair, so much so that her family has lost more than 600 pounds. Over the years she constantly gained weight courtesy, she says, of frequenting "All You Can Eat" buffets until her 5-foot, 3-inch frame was carrying a 232-pound burden, and walking up a flight of stairs to her office used to take her fifteen to twenty minutes.

Coincidentally, she heard about The Micro Diet within hours of one of the most embarrassing experiences of her life when her younger brother, the Reverend Mike Hodge, was being ordained. "I went to church wearing my size thirty-eight men's stretch pants—with the top button undone—because I didn't have a dress that would fit me," says Beverly. "I was the only woman there in pants and tried to hide by sitting on the back row. Then they asked his entire family to go up front and stand with him while the church welcomed him. Standing there in front of everybody, I thought I would die of embarrassment. I felt knee-high to a duck."

That same evening Beverly saw a sixty-second television commercial for The Micro Diet and made a call which, she says, changed her life. Still somewhat skeptical after a lifetime of trying different ways to lose weight, she asked three doctors their opinion of The Micro Diet. Each of them approved. Beverly quickly began to approve, too, losing fifty-three pounds in thirteen weeks. She thought that was remarkable, compared with her experience visiting a storefront weight-loss center. "I spent fifteen hundred dollars and lost only fourteen pounds in four months, and the people there thought that was good. I said, 'you've got to be kidding.'"

Beverly has now lost a total of seventy-two pounds and wants to get rid of another twenty-five. Her success has inspired other members of her family. Daughter Marilyn Byram has lost 140 pounds, and kept if off for a year. Daughter Jackie and son-in-law Steve have together lost over 100 pounds and also maintained for a year. Brother Gary Hodge lost forty-six pounds and his wife twenty-nine pounds, and not regained for over two years. And the rest of the family line-up—Sister Sue Mayfield has lost thirty-five pounds and her son, Mike, twenty-five; granddaughter kala Smith, (forty pounds), sister Colleen Hearon (twenty-five pounds), aunt

Thelma Williams (thirty-five pounds), niece Elaine Edwards (twenty-five pounds), and mother-in-law, Lillian Smith, (twenty-five pounds).

Says Beverly, "My whole family is involved because of me. I remember arriving at a funeral once and two people having to help me out of the car, I was so big and unhealthy. All of my relatives know what kind of condition I was in back then, and have witnessed the transformation in me, so I guess I'm the role model." Their support system was obviously their own family. "We always support each other, so helping each other with the diet just came naturally. We're in frequent contact all the time, so I'm able to make sure everyone's doing O.K. When someone loses five pounds, I'm as happy as they are," says Beverly.

"I usually talk to my daughter Jackie every day to see how she's doing, and I stay on top of Marilyn all the time. She used to be so big that she wore forty-six-inch stretch pants that were as tight as can be. I also keep in regular touch with aunt Thelma in Oklahoma and Gary calls me from everywhere."

And these days, Beverly doesn't have a problem when it comes to thinking of Christmas presents—she gives members of her family their favorite Micro Diet meal with a note saying, "This is my gift of life to you from me."

We have known all along the immense value to the program of our Advisor network. It was proven in the University of Surrey survey of dieters, with 77% describing the role of the Advisor as "important" or "fairly important."

Jacqueline Stordy, who conducted that survey, agrees that such support is critical. Writing in a publication for doctors, she bluntly told them, "The doctor has to decide who should give the advice—themselves, a dietitian, slimming club leader, or lay advisor. Whoever gives the advice, the dieter needs empathy and regular contact outside clinic or office hours.

"Doctors and dietitians may find the most efficient and effective way to provide empathy and support is for them to liaise closely with lay advisors or slimming club leaders. Empathy is sometimes missing in care. A real understanding of the difficulty of dietary restraint in the face of friends, family, colleagues, and a plentiful supply of palatable food is required. Such sympathy is often most easily provided by people who themselves have a weight problem they have sought to resolve."

Eminent authorities in the field have also now concluded that such support is an essential part of a successful weight-loss regimen. Dr. Denis Craddock reported in the British Medical Association Slimmer's Guide: "For those who have difficulty in keeping to a diet, groups run by hospitals, family doctors, local authorities, and slimming organizations can be valuable."

Professor Stunkard, of the University of Pennsylvania, stated in a scientific paper: "We could make the treatment of obesity more extensive by applying behavioral methods to large populations through the agency of lay-led groups."

Dr. Stunkard also recommends a method that The Micro Diet has employed with great effect—friendly competition. He says, "Competition, particularly between different work sites, has proven to be a powerful motivation for weight loss."

Dr. Stunkard told an international conference on obesity that in a normal weight-loss program of 175 participants there was a drop-out rate of 34% and an average weight loss of 7.3 pounds. When rival teams were set up (three banks competing against each other) the drop-out rate plummeted to 0.5% and weight loss was almost twice as good—thirteen pounds average over a twelve-week period. Team spirit was the overriding factor, with members not wishing to let each other down. Such competition, he said, was also instrumental in encouraging men to participate in losing weight.

In Great Britain and New Zealand, The Micro Diet, in conjunction with national newspapers, organized "Slimming Olympics," with large cash prizes as an added incentive. Hundreds of groups got together to battle it out for the gold medals. The British winning team was comprised of six homemakers who between them lost 120 pounds in six weeks, an average of twenty pounds each. The runners-up were six nurses (101 pounds), and six hairdressers (eighty-six pounds).

The Micro Diet in Great Britain also helped raise funds for a children's charity by promoting an event in which dieters were sponsored by family, friends, and acquaintances and collected donations per pound lost. Some American researchers have also been looking at this technique as a means of improving weight loss.

## *THE MULTI-PRONGED ATTACK*

Several studies published in the *Journal of the American Dietetic Association* have focused on the benefits of a multi-pronged approach to weight control involving nutrition education, exercise, behavioral changes, and support.

In one study of over 2,000 people conducted at the Kaiser Permanente Center for Health Research in Portland, Oregon, participants attended weekly meetings as long as they wished and were encouraged to maintain food diaries to monitor and control their eating pattern. One of the key findings was that adults of all ages and weights can be comfortably mixed in a support group. Those members who are already succeeding in losing weight serve as motivational role models for newcomers—a common occurrence experienced at Micro Diet meetings.

The workplace can often be an ideal location for a weight management program, not only because it's obviously a convenient meeting place, but also because of the constant support from coworkers and supervisors. A report prepared by the Dairy Council of Arizona says, "Employers are usually enthusiastic about implementing the programs after being shown that weight loss may increase productivity, improve company morale, and decrease employee sick time. Employee/management relations also seem to improve as a result of the increased communication."

The success of a study involving twenty employees at the corporate headquarters of a major supermarket chain was primarily attributed to the dieters' active involvement in planning their own weight-loss program. They identified behaviors that led to their overeating, and they implemented changes, and designed exercise programs for themselves based on their own capabilities and goals.

## *LASTING RESULTS*

Let's be honest. Losing excess weight is one thing, maintaining that weight loss is an entirely different matter. The long-term failure rate is quite extraordinary. All of the available evidence indicates that diet support and behavior modification (including an exercise program) are essential ingredients of permanent success.

In a major overview published in *Behavior Therapy*, Dr. Kelly Brownell, of the University of Pennsylvania, and Dr. Robert Jeffrey of the University of Minnesota, challenged the complacent attitude of many behavior therapists, and declared, "It is time to be daring and innovative... new and aggressive methods must be proposed if we are to have a significant impact on the problem of obesity."

In their article entitled "Improving Long-Term Weight Loss: Pushing the Limits of Treatment," these two prominent psychiatrists enthused, "Exciting results have come recently from using behavior therapy with very low-calorie diets and from the use of behavioral programs in work sites."

One of the studies which impressed them, which was carried out at the same university, compared the effectiveness of: a very low-calorie diet alone; behavior therapy alone; and very low-calorie diet, plus behavior therapy. The combined method produced significantly greater weight losses at both the end of treatment (forty-two-and-a-half pounds—eleven pounds more than the other methods) and at follow-up one year later (twenty-eight pounds). The patients who participated in the behavior change program regained only one-third of their weight loss while the diet-only group regained two-thirds.

Cautioning that rapid weight loss can be followed by rapid weight regain, the researchers feel "these results...add to the increasing evidence of the effectiveness of behavior therapy. Further research is needed to improve the application of behavior therapy to very low-calorie diet."

When the same group of dieters was followed up after three years, it was found that 19% of those individuals receiving a combined treatment had maintained a weight loss within five pounds of their end-of-treatment loss, compared with 13% of the "diet alone" group, and just 7% of those participating in behavior therapy alone.

After three years, the "diet alone" group, who had lost an average of 31 pounds at the end of treatment, had maintained a weight loss of 8¼ pounds. For the behavior therapy patients the respective figures were 31½ pounds and 10½ pounds and for the combined group, 42½ pounds and 14½ pounds. The value of the behavior therapy treatment, therefore, did seem to diminish over time. Subjects in all three conditions had regained between 74% and 85% of their original weight loss. Anecdotally, the researchers heard that many of the successful dieters had not practiced the weight control methods in which they had been instructed.

Some of the dieters had enrolled in additional treatment and lost weight again, lending credence to the fact that weight maintenance is a lifelong struggle. The researchers reported "repeated weight control efforts may prove fruitful." Unfortunately, it appears that the dieters waited too long—until they had virtually regained all of their lost weight before seeking further help.

This provides support for the experts who have even gone so far as to suggest that obesity should be regarded as an incurable, chronic disease and, therefore, behavior change sessions "should never be abandoned." Baylor College of Medicine researchers G. K. Goodrick and J. P. Foreyt have suggested that for long-term success, the dieter should seriously consider attending lifetime "booster" sessions.

In conclusion, I have to stress the value of support, particularly from someone who, as Dr. Stordy says, can empathize with the dieter, someone who has been along the same road. In numerous letters and at many meetings I've been told countless times: "I couldn't have made it without my Advisor," or "I was really depressed, and then The Micro Diet meeting gave me all my enthusiasm back."

The Advisors come from all walks of life: nurses and dietitians, for example, who can provide additional insight into the medical and nutritional aspects; but also homemakers, secretaries, business executives, engineers, and factory workers. In England, all of British society has been represented. There's a baroness and a shepherdess, even a millionaire. And now an ever-growing network in the U.S. of doctors, nurses, pharmacists, homemakers, lawyers, insurance brokers, stock brokers—truly, people from all walks of life.

## ■ A CASE STUDY

### SUZANNE DEBLANC: NOW MORE THAN A "PRETTY FACE"

Suzanne DeBlanc's children gave her the incentive to finally tackle her weight problem. "My oldest had just started kindergarten and, knowing how cruel children can be, I didn't want to be known as 'the fat mother,'" says the thirty-two-year-old mother of two, of Houston, Texas. Adds Suzanne, who weighed 280 pounds before she started The Micro Diet, "I also came to realize that I'm responsible for two other lives, and I didn't want my kids to grow up to be as big as me."

Suzanne now feels the strong need to motivate her children from an early age to adopt sensible eating behavior and an exercise routine. "Let's be real: most habits are learned in the home, so I've changed for the kids. This is a family thing and I'm leading by example."

Suzanne lays the blame for gaining weight plainly and squarely on her eating habits, especially during her own childhood growing up in the south where heavy fried food and rich sauces were the order of the day. Candy such as Snickers and Milky Way bars were also part of her downfall. "Stock in both those companies went down when I started The Micro Diet," she says with a laugh.

Suzanne, a yo-yo dieter, experienced her share of ridicule and discrimination when she was overweight. She often heard people say, "You have such a pretty face, but..." Even though she has a B.S. in management, a previous boss took her to one side to tell her, "You won't go very far unless you lose some weight." Says Suzanne, "People would talk down to me as if I was stupid because of my weight."

There's no way that that happens today. So far, Suzanne has lost 111 pounds and wants to get rid of another twenty-nine pounds. It's the first time in her life that she has had such success. "I have literally been on everything, and the most I've every lost before was forty pounds, and that was when I was virtually starving myself. I would eat nothing and then have a diet pop and popcorn feast for a couple of days. What attracted me to The Micro Diet was that the food was good, the cost wasn't prohibitive, and an Advisor contacted me in my own home. That made a big difference. Both Weight Watchers and Opti-Fast make you weigh in in front of someone. I did not like that. That's something I want to do in the privacy of my own home.

"The Micro Diet makes me feel like I'm in control. The message I got from some of those other programs was 'burn in hell' if you didn't comply with their way of doing things. I was so desperate before The Micro Diet that I was even looking into getting my stomach stapled. We are talking major surgery. The whole process is very uncomfortable and I know I was trying to buy willpower because I felt I didn't have it myself."

Suzanne lost twenty-nine pounds her first month on The Micro Diet and believes that rapid rate of loss provided her with the motivation she needed to continue. That success made her attentive to all of the other recommendations in The Micro Diet program and she now chooses foods more wisely and exercises five times a week.

Suzanne speaks highly of the Advisor support system. "My Advisor was a great emotional support. I didn't need someone's shoulders to cry on, but we would talk at least once a week. She would ask me specific questions about how I was doing and offer suggestions so I wouldn't get bored. It's nice to have someone who will follow through."

# 11

# NOT FOR WEIGHT LOSS ONLY

THE LOSER-FRIENDLY MICRO DIET is not just a weight-loss program—it's a way of life. The nutritious meals are ideal for anyone who cares about maintaining his or her ideal weight, or obtaining proper nutrition. For growing children, they are a perfect high-nutrition snack. For athletes, or anyone with an active lifestyle, they are a superb nutritional supplement. For the elderly, who so often are at risk of malnutrition, they are convenient, easy-to-prepare nutrition-rich meals.

All of the essential nutrients—especially the *micro* nutrients, the vitamins, minerals, trace elements, and electrolytes—are found in specific, measured amounts in every Micro meal. Most of our kitchens today are stocked with ready-to-eat meals, so why not choose easy-to-fix meals that provide you with complete balanced nutrition and have a shelf life of six to eighteen months? After all, your body is more complex than the most sophisticated computer, and requires the entire nutritional alphabet of nutrients—often interacting—to perform a wide variety of tasks.

These nutrients—from vitamin A to zinc—have to:

(a) furnish the fuel,
(b) build and maintain body tissues, and
(c) regulate body processes.

They're all provided in The Micro Diet. Three to four Micro

meals provide at least 100% of the recommended amounts of all necessary nutrients. By contrast, many people who try to lose weight by simply cutting back on their caloric intake also cut back on their nutritional intake, with the result that they may be deficient in certain vital nutrients. And people who elect to go to a fast food restaurant are now well aware of the nutritional disasters that await them there.

Most people can obtain all of the nutrients they need by eating a diet rich in vegetables, fruits, meats, and dairy products. But most people, in reality, no matter how "aware" they might be, are nowhere near accomplishing that. It just doesn't fit into their lifestyle or eating habits.

For instance, Kathryn Collins, M.D., a fourteen-year emergency room veteran, faces intense, unpredictable workdays, between ten and fourteen hours long. In her demanding schedule she is often lucky to get a ten-minute meal break. That's where the loser-friendly Micro Diet appealed to her. She wanted to lose fifteen pounds—a feat she accomplished. But the big attraction was the convenience and nutritional profile of the meals.

Says Dr. Collins, of Dubuque, Iowa, "This is not just for weight loss. The meals are nutritionally balanced, they provide the perfect fast food. I know many health professionals as well as patients who use it like I do as a quick, easy meal replacement. It's ideally suited for the elderly from the nutritional standpoint. I see lots of malnutrition in the elderly because many of them can't take care of themselves. The Micro Diet is easy for them because it requires little preparation time and gives them that complete balanced nutrition."

Family practitioner, James Webber, M.D., a "womb to tomb" physician, as he describes himself, is a firm believer in preventive medicine, and the need for everyone to obtain proper nutrition.

"I recommend that my patients have three Micro meals a day. By doing this I feel they are very secure in their nutrition. Since I've been recommending this system to parents, I've found that their children are using the meals, too, and eating a lot less junk foods. I feel much more confident that these children are getting the nutrition that they need. The athletes that I have in my practice are also benefitting, as most of them are interested in gaining strength, endurance, and stamina without accumulating extra fat. Even bodybuilders have benefitted from what I call 'micro fuel.' They look at it as a system whereby they can add muscle bulk without excessive body fat.

"The program provides the working patient with an inexpensive, low-fat diet that allows them to nourish themselves quickly, conveniently, and efficiently. Speaking for myself, as a doctor I had a very difficult time nourishing myself throughout the day. Most of the time I would go all day without eating, even though I knew it was a bad idea. The Micro Diet provided me with a very easy way to obtain good nutrition. The meals are so simple to prepare and I've never felt better."

Every single Micro meal serves carefully measured amounts of ALL known micro nutrients—at least 35% of the U.S. government's Recommended Dietary Allowance (RDA). It is absolutely no use consuming megadoses of one nutrient only to be deficient in another, equally important, nutrient. To achieve this remarkable nutritional package in so few calories by selecting food from supermarket shelves would be a daunting task for the most experienced nutritionist. With The Micro Diet it just couldn't be simpler.

The "first wave" of vitamin research in the early part of the 20th century was the actual discovery of vitamins and their ability to combat nutritional deficiencies such as rickets and beriberi, and the results are indisputable. The "second wave"—the claims that heavier doses of certain nutrients are necessary for optimal health and the prevention of some chronic disease—is today a hotly debated issue.

Although 40%–60% of Americans take some kind of nutritional supplement, a report from the National Research Council, issued in 1989, bluntly stated that a good health recommendation was to avoid taking supplements in excess of the RDA. The 1,300-page volume—the result of a three-year study—declared, "Vitamin-mineral supplements that exceed the RDA...not only have no known health benefits...but their use may be detrimental to health."

Dr. Arno Motulsky, a University of Washington professor who was chairman of the NRC committee, said that while such supplements, "may make people feel better, the evidence that this helps prevent chronic disease is nonexistent. Having no evidence of scientific benefits, we don't recommend it."

Since that report, however, there has been growing acceptance in the scientific community that higher doses of some nutrients may play an important role in protecting against a wide range of maladies. It is beginning to appear as if the "traditional" view may have been short-sighted.

Since the 1970s, in fact, worldwide surveys have been consistently uncovering a link between diet and health and, more recently, the focus has been on the beneficial properties of specific vitamins and minerals. In particular, there has been considerable attention paid to the antioxidants, vitamins C, E, and beta carotene, the chemical parent of vitamin A. What do they do? Well, in effect, they fight against "killer" molecules known as free radicals which, it is thought, injure and destroy DNA and various body cells leading to the development of cancer, heart and lung disease, and cataracts. Antioxidants are being heralded in some quarters as having the potential for breakthrough improvements in health care.

Here's a brief review of the A to Z of nutrition, all of which is provided for you in Micro meals.

## *PROTEIN*

Protein provides the twenty-two different amino acids that build our bodies and tissues. Of these, eight are called "essential" (nine for infants) because the body cannot make them: they have to come from the food we eat. Every single body cell contains protein: the skin, teeth and nails, hair and bones. As these body proteins are continuously broken down, and some protein is lost, the body's protein stores have to be constantly replenished.

If you read the tables produced by most governments, you will find some variation in the average amount of protein recommended. The U.S. government recommends an average of fifty-six grams for men and forty-four grams for women. That assumes a mixed diet of both high-quality and low-quality protein, and is increased to account for individual variations.

## *CARBOHYDRATE*

A primary function of digestible carbohydrate is to serve as a major source of energy for the body. All of the nutrients work together to promote a healthy body and this is particularly true of carbohydrate and protein. Carbohydrate operates hand in glove with protein to make the action of the protein more efficient. If there were not enough carbohydrate in the diet, the body would break down protein to provide carbohydrate for the brain to use, "stealing" protein from its main purpose of repairing tissues and promoting growth. Digestible carbohydrates also promote normal fat metabolism and help prevent loss of sodium.

## *FAT*

Fat in the diet is necessary to provide the essential fatty acids, but it does "cost" nine calories per gram or 252 calories per ounce, so we need enough, but not too much.

## *SODIUM/POTASSIUM/CHLORIDE*

These three electrolytes interact to keep body cells functioning properly. In balanced proportions they are essential for muscle and nerve activity. They also help acid balance of body fluids. A deficiency can cause tiredness and irregular heartbeats. Sodium chloride is the chemical name given to common salt, so foods rich in this condiment—such as processed and preserved products—are also high in sodium and chloride. Potassium is present in most common foods in moderate amounts. Fruit and vegetables (particularly potatoes and bananas), and instant coffee are rich sources. It is worth noting, however, that too much sodium may cause water retention and hypertension. Some people are particularly sensitive to excessive salt in their diet.

## *CALCIUM/PHOSPHORUS*

Calcium and phosphorus build strong bones and teeth. Calcium is especially important for expectant mothers, children, and people susceptible to osteoporosis (brittle bones). These nutrients need the help of vitamin D to be effective. The most valuable sources of calcium are milk and cheese. However, beans and other vegetables also contribute calcium to the diet. In general, rich food sources of calcium are also rich in phosphorus.

## *MAGNESIUM*

Magnesium is essential for all living cells for the functioning of some of the enzymes involved in energy utilization. It helps keep muscles working. Most natural foods contain useful amounts of magnesium; cereals and vegetables make particularly valuable contributions.

## *IRON*

Iron keeps your blood healthy. It forms part of the red pigments of blood, which carries oxygen from your lungs to every part of your body and takes the waste product, carbon dioxide, back to your lungs. Meat is a good source of iron.

## *ZINC*

This trace element is required for growth, wound healing, skin health, and resistance to infection. Good dietary sources in daily use are meats, legumes, and whole grains.

## *COPPER*

Copper is an essential trace element which forms part of many enzyme systems. Its metabolism in the body is closely related to that of iron. Deficiency causes anemia. Green vegetables, many species of fish, oysters, and liver are all good sources of copper, but most other foods provide only small amounts.

## *MANGANESE*

This is a trace element associated with a number of enzymes. Deficiency causes poor growth and bone deformities in animals. Rich providers of manganese are whole cereals, legumes, and leafy vegetables.

## *MOLYBDENUM*

A trace element which forms a vital part of several enzyme systems, molybdenum may help prevent tooth decay. Among the best sources of molybdenum are cabbage, carrots, potatoes, and broad beans.

## *IODINE*

Iodine is vital to the metabolism. It contributes to the hormones thyroxine and triiodothyronine, which help regulate metabolic rate. Fish and iodized salt are rich sources. Fruits, vegetables, cereals, and meat provide varying amounts of iodine.

## *FAT-SOLUBLE VITAMINS*

### Vitamin A

Vitamin A is essential for vision in dim light and for the maintenance of healthy skin, eyes and hair, and surface tissue in general. There are growing claims that beta carotene, the chemical parent of Vitamin A, may reduce the risk of breast, lung, colon, and cervical cancer, as well as heart disease and stroke. It is found mainly in milk, butter, cheese, egg yolks, liver, and some fatty fish. However, carotenes can be converted into Vitamin A in the body and rich sources of these pigments include carrots, leafy vegetables, and apricots.

### Vitamin D

This vitamin is actually manufactured in the skin when exposed to sunlight. By far the richest dietary source are fish liver oils. Milk and orange juice are also fortified with vitamin D, which is required for strong teeth and bone and has been shown to prevent rickets. It maintains the level of calcium and phosphorus in the blood. It has been suggested that it also may prevent osteoporosis and kidney disease.

### Vitamin E

Vitamin E is believed to serve a function in keeping blood cells healthy and it does counteract rancidity in fats. It has been claimed that Vitamin E may also reduce the risk of angina and heart attack. The best sources are vegetable oils and, therefore, margarine and shortening also provide considerable amounts.

### Vitamin K

It has long been established that Vitamin K is necessary for the normal clotting of blood. Now it appears that Vitamin K helps bones retain calcium. A recent Dutch study of 1,500 women revealed that calcium loss was cut in half with daily Vitamin K supplementation. You can seek to get enough by eating fresh leafy vegetables as well as cereals, dairy products, meats, and fruits.

## *WATER-SOLUBLE VITAMINS*

### Vitamin C

Necessary for healthy connective tissue, teeth, gums, and bones, Vitamin C also builds strong body cells and blood vessels. It is also possible, according to one Canadian study, that high doses of Vitamin C (and Vitamin E) may deter the development of cataracts. Another fascinating paper in 1992, in the journal *Epidemiology*, reported on a 10-year study of 11,000 adults and found that those consuming higher doses of vitamin C lived longer. Men who consumed about 300 milligrams a day from food and supplements suffered 41% fewer deaths during the study than those with the lowest intake (less than fifty milligrams a day). Fresh fruit and green leafy vegetables are excellent sources of this vitamin. Potatoes are not a particularly good source but as large amounts may be eaten they can be the major provider of Vitamin C.

### Thiamine/Vitamin B1

This is required for the steady and continuous release of energy from carbohydrates. A deficiency of this vitamin produces beriberi. Brewers yeast and bran are good providers of thiamine.

### Riboflavin/Vitamin B2

Riboflavin is necessary for healthy skin, and building and maintaining body tissues. It is also concerned with the sensitivity of the eyes to light and required for the releasing of energy from food. It is found in significant amounts in liver, milk, eggs, and green vegetables but, in contrast to other B vitamins, it is relatively lacking in cereal grains.

### Pyridoxine/Vitamin B6

This nutrient is involved in the metabolism of amino acids. It is necessary for the formation of hemoglobin and the proper functioning of the nervous system. It helps prevent anemia, skin lesions, and nerve damage. Good providers include liver, whole grain cereals, peanuts, and bananas, but most foods are moderate sources.

## Niacin

Required to convert food to energy, aid the nervous system, and to maintain a healthy skin. Humans do not rely totally on dietary intake of this vitamin as it may also be synthesized from tryptophan, one of the essential amino acids.

## Pantothenic Acid

Pantothenic acid is necessary for the release of energy from fat and carbohydrate. It is also required for tissue growth. The richest sources of pantothenic acid include liver, kidney, yeast, bran, and egg yolk.

## Folic Acid

In conjunction with B12, folic acid is highly necessary for healthy blood formation, and is important in tissues where cells are dividing rapidly, e.g., during pregnancy. It is also possible that folic acid can help prevent children from being born with crippling neurological defects such as spina bifida (incomplete closure of the spine) and anencephaly, in which the brain does not fully develop. A British study showed that when women who had already given birth to one handicapped child received folic acid supplements during a subsequent pregnancy, their chances of producing a healthy baby rose dramatically.

Another tantalizing report from the University of Alabama revealed that women exposed to a virus that causes cervical cancer were five times more likely to develop precancerous lesions if they had low blood levels of folic acid. Found in liver, kidney, spinach, and broccoli tops, folic acid can be deficient in the diets of many people, particularly the poor.

## Biotin

Essential for the metabolism of fat. The richest sources are liver, kidney, and yeast extract, but many species of bacteria can make or retain biotin, so humans can probably obtain all they need from micro-organisms in food and in the gut.

## Vitamin B12

Working with folic acid, vitamin B12 is essential for healthy blood formation and the nervous system. It is only found in foods of animal origin.

### ■ A CASE STUDY

### ED RICKARDS: CANCEL THOSE FUNERAL ARRANGEMENTS

"I couldn't have done it without my extraordinary network of Micro Diet Advisors," says retired food service manager Edmund Rickards. "Having this direct line to others who have struggled with their weight led to my victory." Sixty-four-year-old Ed lost eighty-three pounds in five-and-a-half months and, at 235 pounds, weighs ten pounds less than he did at age sixteen.

"I worked for over forty years in the food industry and my life revolved around food, and lots of it," he says. Then, in May 1990, weighing 321 pounds, Ed moved to Palm Desert, California, "to literally spend my last days in the sun. I could hardly walk upstairs, my health was ailing and, worst of all, I was resigned to remain this way. My wife and I even made funeral arrangements, we were so convinced I didn't have long to live."

Then he saw The Micro Diet on a television show. "There was an entire audience of successful dieters who used to look and feel like I did. That was all the motivation I needed. As my weight decreased, my energy increased, and a brand-new future of hope and opportunity opened up before me."

Just how important was the Advisor support? "I would have given up after two weeks if it hadn't been for the support of my Advisor, Nancy Murray. She told me I could call her anytime. Well, I did call her once at 7 A.M. On another occasion I was disgusted and very discouraged because I had reached a plateau. So I called Nancy and she suggested I keep a chart of what I ate during the week to see what the problem was. This chart helped me realize just how much I nibbled here and there while cooking or baking, and enabled me to get back on a weight-loss track," says Ed. "For me, it is the Advisor support that makes The Micro Diet special. Some programs claim to provide support but a once-a-week meeting doesn't cut it for me."

Ed used to attend one organization's weekly meetings, and says, "I needed support more often than that. If I needed some help I couldn't afford to wait for the next meeting, especially when I knew it meant being weighed in front of everybody else. You know someone is going to end up weighing the most and it seemed that person was always me. By contrast, The Micro Diet is such a non-judgmental program. I can't believe the energy I now have. I'm a new man."

Ed, in fact, has so much energy that he now works as a hospital volunteer three times a week, as well as helping other people with their weight problems. "My attitude is that I'll take calls any time of day or night. I've been helped, and I feel very strongly about providing others with the same kind of support. Having maintained his weight loss for over a year, Ed is thrilled with his "new life." "I am walking, living proof that The Micro Diet is not just for those who wish to lose weight, but for those who are ready to live a happier and healthier life."

Ed avoided exercise all of his life until a Micro Diet Advisor persuaded him of the error of his ways. "I was able to get through high school without ever taking a gym class because I would get my doctor to write a medical excuse." In his adult life, he says, "I've worn out more easy chairs than I care to say." He would go shopping with his wife, only to make a point of finding the nearest chair and flopping into it.

After watching Ed's successful weight loss, an Advisor persistently encouraged him to start exercising until Ed finally agreed to give it a try. "I started walking about two blocks and then gradually I increased the amount every week until I reached a mile and a half. I'm doing it three times a week and it has made a big difference in the way I feel. I now substitute walking for all the times I would take the lazy man's way out. I no longer use my wife's disability card to park up front. I park farther away and walk."

# 12

# THE EXCELLENCE OF EXERCISE

WHEN YOU'RE OVERWEIGHT and the sheer effort of carrying around those excess pounds is hard enough, just the thought of deliberate physical exertion can make you feel tired enough to collapse into the nearest chair. Do you have to exercise to lose weight? Just how important is exercise? What's the best kind?

Well, you don't have to exercise to lose weight, but exercise is vitally important in helping you lose more fat than lean body tissue, and exercise will make it much easier to keep the weight off. And "exercise" doesn't mean you're going to be asked to vigorously perform a one-hour Jane Fonda workout "going for the burn." You'll get started with simple lifestyle exercises.

First, let's make it very clear: To lose weight you must cut back on your food intake. Exercise by itself—without a diet program—is not very effective, especially when large losses are desired within a relatively short time period. Weekly losses from a diet program alone are often ten times greater than losses due to an exercise program alone.

Several studies have shown, however, that exercise has a valuable role to play in preservation of fat-free mass. One study compared seventy-two mildly obese members of the Boston Police Department who were divided into "diet and exercise" and "diet-only" groups. Although there was little difference in weight, the exercisers lost a significanty greater proportion of FAT.

In another study eight obese women were placed on 800 calories a day for five weeks. Five of them took part in a daily progressive walking program: the other three did no exercise at all. There was no significant difference in weight loss, but considerable difference in fat loss. The dieters who exercised lost 74% of their weight from fat; the non-exercisers just 57%.

Does it matter what kind of exercise? A University of Wisconsin–Madison study compared the effect of high- and low-intensity workouts with a group of twenty-seven overweight women.

All of the women were placed on a 1,200-calorie-a-day program for eight weeks and assigned either a high or low work rate, three days a week on a cycle ergometer. There was no difference in the amount of weight lost or the composition of body mass, i.e., fat or lean body tissue. Of significance, however, was the fact that the dieters on the high-intensity regimen had a much harder time performing at the desired level, especially at the beginning. The high-intensity group experienced labored breathing and had to split the exercise into two or more segments, leading researchers to recommend, at least initially, a low-intensity program in combination with diet.

And what about exercise in conjunction with a very low-calorie diet? Researchers at the University of Cambridge set up a test in which they followed sixty overweight women who were consuming just 405 calories per day for eight weeks, followed by eight weeks on a maintenance program of 1,500 calories per day. Some of the dieters participated in aerobic exercise on bicycle machines; others did isotonic resistance exercises, while others did six weeks of one kind of exercise and eight weeks of the other. Two other groups followed the respective exercise programs but did not diet.

Very similar patterns of weight loss were observed in the "dieting only" and "dieting plus exercise" groups. "Exercise only" groups achieved slight weight gains. The researchers commented, "The results of this study indicate that controlled aerobic and isotonic resistance training can be undertaken and sustained during periods of weight reduction using a very low-calorie diet."

In other words, drastically reducing one's caloric intake doesn't handicap your physical performance as long as it's exercise of moderate intensity. You can do it.

Other research has indicated that the duration and frequency of exercise is more important than intensity—four times a week promoted markedly greater weight loss than twice weekly.

The most important role of exercise is in the **maintenance** of weight loss. One study of thirteen middle-aged men showed a 22% loss in body fat during thirty-five weeks of marathon training. Seven men discontinued training; six continued at a reduced level. Eight weeks later the body fat levels of those who had stopped training had returned to 95% of their pretraining levels. The men who had continued training had no increase at all. Another study showed that 80%–90% of people who had never been overweight had consistently exercised.

A major review of long-term approaches to weight maintenance came to the unequivocal conclusion that a regular exercise program is critical. Dr. Daniel J. Safer, of the Johns Hopkins University School of Medicine, writing in the *Southern Medical Journal,* commented on "a prominent association between continued exercise and comparative success in maintaining weight loss." In one study, seventeen obese adults who exercised regularly maintained a thirty pound average weight loss over a fifteen-month follow-up period. By contrast, program participants who did not exercise regained an average of 40% of their lost weight.

In another study it was reported that eleven of the thirteen men and seventeen of the forty-one women who maintained their weight loss for an average of six years exercised vigorously and consistently, more than thirty minutes, three to five times a week.

Says Dr. Safer, "In addition to the weight-loss benefits of exercise for the obese, a large amount of evidence indicates that mild to moderate exercise by itself (and often in conjunction with a diet) has a broad range of other health advantages. Exercise improves self-concept and mood, improves fitness, increases lean muscle mass, decreases body fat, blood cholesterol, plasma insulin, and blood pressure, and maintains the basal metabolic rate at a customary level during dieting."

Prominent researcher Edward S. Horton, M.D., chairman of the Department of Medicine at the University of Vermont, agrees. "As part of a weight-control program exercise is of great importance, particularly because it has now been shown in a number of studies to be the single most important factor in long-term maintenance. The combination of a low-calorie intake and increased energy expenditure through physical activity is the most effective way to *achieve* weight loss and *maintain* weight loss.

"Exercise increases the amount of fat loss and tends to preserve the lean body mass, the muscle mass. Regular exercise also increases cardiovascular function. It decreases the risk factors associated with high cholesterol and high lipid levels. The specific effects of a regular exercise program are to lower the triglyceride levels in the blood and to increase the HDL cholesterol, the so-called 'good cholesterol.'

"Exercise also results in a lowering of blood pressure in people who have mild to moderate hypertension, and it increases insulin sensitivity and tends to lower blood glucose, so it is a very important factor in preventing the development of non-insulin dependent diabetes in people with obesity."

The best kind of exercise? Rather than programmed exercise (calisthenics) or apparatus-based workouts, go for a lifestyle exercise program, such as bicycling, stair climbing, or athletic competition, says Dr. Safer. Better still, find a "social" program. There's a threefold lower drop-out rate for those participating in groups rather than going it alone. So don't wake up in the morning and ask yourself, "Do I really have to exercise today?" Know that the answer is YES and make sure you do it. After all, the inescapable energy equation is that:

| Calories Eaten | Minus | Calories burnt for work or keeping warm | = Weight gain or loss |
|---|---|---|---|

If you eat 2,200 calories and only use 2,000 calories, you gain 200 calories which is stored mostly as fat. You certainly wouldn't notice it. If you continued each day, it would be 1,400 calories extra stored as fat in the course of a week. Still not noticeable. But by continuing on that course for a month, you would gain nearly one and a half pounds (because 3,500 excess calories equals one pound of body fat). Still no real apparent problem.

But what would happen if you continued to eat an extra 200 calories each day for a year? You wouldn't continue to gain at the rate of one and a half pounds every month, because the body adapts to excess caloric intake in two ways: 1) the excess intake stimulates the metabolic rate which burns off some of the extra calories and, 2) as you gain weight your total daily energy expenditure increases because of your larger body size. This means that eventually you would be burning 2,200 calories per day rather than your original 2,000 calories. Therefore, if you continued to take in an extra 200 calories a day you would gain weight until a new state of energy balance was achieved. In most people this would be after a gain of ten to fifteen pounds.

As if to add insult to injury, as people put on weight they also tend to become slower and less active, a trend that cars, and all the modern labor-saving devices accentuate. What's more, the less active you are, the more tired you tend to feel, and inactivity actually leads you to eat more than you would with a more active lifestyle. Furthermore, as you get older you experience a decline in your metabolic rate!

But here's some good news: we burn a certain number of calories doing absolutely nothing. It's called your "basal metabolic rate" or "resting metabolic rate." So even when you're lying in bed doing nothing, energy is still required for your heart to pump blood around your system and for the body's other biochemical processes—about 1,000 to 2,000 calories a day. (Your heart has to pump blood through 59,520 miles of capillaries, veins, and arteries, enough to wind around the earth twice.) The basal metabolic rate is dependent upon body size but for someone, for example, maintaining weight on about 2,500 calories a day, about 1,500 calories will be expended as part of the basal metabolic rate. One can burn up to 900 calories a day simply moving around a room, or even fidgeting.

The second piece of good news is that you also burn calories digesting the food you've consumed. The thermic effect of food is what happens for a few hours after a meal when the rate of energy expenditure increases to absorb and process the food. On average it is about five to ten percent of calories consumed. So if you eat 2,500 calories a day, you can count on "automatically" losing up to 250 calories of it through the effort involved digesting it.

By being physically active, however, you're going to burn considerably more calories. The highest daily rates of energy expenditure that have ever been measured were of competitors in the Tour de France bicycle race, an average of a staggering 4,000 to 5,000 calories a day. But that, of course, is only over a limited period.

Says Dr. Horton, "The average amount of energy expenditure from physical activity can, therefore, vary enormously from as low as 300–500 calories a day up to, in very extreme conditions, as much as 4,000–5,000 calories a day."

## *GETTING STARTED*

So now you want to exercise? Right? So where do you start? Be warned. Most people give up on exercise because, once they have made the commitment, they throw themselves wholeheartedly into it. They try to do too much, too soon. You don't have to force yourself through a rigorous, exhausting routine. You don't have to torture yourself for maximum benefit. Waking up those sleeping muscles doesn't have to be a painful experience. You can do it step-by-step—sometimes literally.

Little changes add up. For instance, if you added ten minutes of walking to your daily schedule, over the course of a year you would burn an additional 14,600 calories. Sure, it doesn't put you in the league of a Tour de France cyclist, but without changing your diet you would lose four pounds.

What's the best exercise *for you?* The best exercise is the one that you will do! The following chart shows you how many calories you burn in ten minutes of activity depending upon your body weight. Notice that in some examples you have the option of easier and harder levels of activity. Highlight the columns for your current weight and your desired weight. (If your weight falls between two weight categories, choose the one closest to your weight.) Think about which of the activities appeal most to you.

If you're like most people, your first inclination is probably to choose the exercise that burns the most calories in the shortest time. Don't do it. On paper, it may appear an attractive proposition but it actually isn't the best choice for burning the most calories or helping you keep faithful to your exercise program.

The keys to successful exercising are: 1) Choose an activity you enjoy; 2) Start at a lower intensity; 3) Begin with a shorter time goal. Have you ever had difficulty staying committed to ice cream? Certainly not, if you enjoy it. Why not apply this enjoyment principle to exercise and keep yourself as firmly committed to exercise as you are currently committed to your favorite foods?

Switching from a sedentary lifestyle to an active one requires a definite attitude adjustment. That's why it is so critical to find one that you will enjoy. Once you discover how much fun exercise can be and once you realize how good it makes you feel, you'll be hooked.

Never lose an opportunity to exercise: you can fit it into your everyday routine. Park at the far side of the office or supermarket

## *CALORIES BURNED IN TEN MINUTES OF ACTIVITY*

| Activity | Weight (pounds) 300 | 250 | 225 | 200 | 175 | 150 | 125 |
|---|---|---|---|---|---|---|---|
| Gardening | 73 | 60 | 54 | 48 | 42 | 36 | 30 |
| Housework | 90 | 76 | 68 | 60 | 53 | 45 | 38 |
| Aerobics (heavy) | 180 | 66 | 60 | 53 | 46 | 40 | 33 |
| Aerobics (light) | 68 | 57 | 51 | 45 | 40 | 34 | 28 |
| Bicycling (6 mph) | 79 | 66 | 60 | 53 | 46 | 40 | 33 |
| Bicycling (10 mph) | 125 | 104 | 94 | 83 | 73 | 62 | 52 |
| Jogging (10 min/mile) | 227 | 189 | 170 | 151 | 132 | 113 | 94 |
| Cross-Country Skiing | 227 | 189 | 170 | 151 | 132 | 113 | 94 |
| Swimming (slow) | 175 | 146 | 131 | 116 | 102 | 87 | 73 |
| Tennis (singles) | 147 | 123 | 111 | 98 | 86 | 73 | 61 |
| Tennis (doubles) | 113 | 94 | 85 | 76 | 66 | 57 | 47 |
| Walking (moderate 20 min/mile) | 79 | 66 | 60 | 53 | 46 | 40 | 33 |
| Walking (easy 26 min/mile) | 68 | 57 | 51 | 45 | 40 | 34 | 28 |

parking lot instead of circling like a vulture, burning up gas looking for a spot closest to the entrance. The extra walk will do you good. If you take the bus, get off a few stops early and enjoy the walk to your destination. Walk up stairs instead of using the elevator. Bend over to put on your shoes without sitting down. Wear comfortable shoes in your spare time, you'll find you walk more. Count everything you do as exercise. When you do housework or yard work put a little extra effort into it.

## *HERE ARE YOUR MARCHING ORDERS*

Get out there—and walk. It's the easiest form of regular exercise to get you back in shape. You don't need any special clothes or equipment. It costs nothing. You can do it everywhere and in almost any weather. It's the ideal way for the overweight person to start exercising and, in fact, in spite of popular belief exercise does not stimulate the appetite, it reduces your desire to eat.

Now, when I say "walking," I don't mean window shopping or a casual stroll. I mean a brisk, sustained walk; a walk into which you put some effort, sufficient to raise your pulse rate. Start out with a one-minute walk. Maybe that sounds a little silly? But it is *getting started* that counts. A one-minute walk is a small goal achievable by everybody. So do it. In reality, of course, you will almost certainly find that you stretch the one minute to five minutes, ten minutes, or more. You have succeeded. Isn't that better than promising yourself that you would exercise for an hour and then failing to take the first step? How many times have you done that? Well, join the club.

Now, technically, sixty minutes is an excellent amount of time to exercise. But starting with sixty minutes is also the perfectionist's path to procrastination. Most people have difficulty finding an hour to spare on exercise—so they never begin. When you try to start with a goal that is too big, you're often overwhelmed by the anticipation alone.

You can bypass the anticipation–procrastination trap by making the one-minute commitment. If after one minute you want to continue, carry on. If you don't, simply return to your other activities and make the one-minute commitment for tomorrow. The important step is the first one: getting off the couch and out the door. Before you know it, the one minute will turn into sixty minutes.

There's another advantage in starting with less exercise and gradually building to a more energetic regimen. If you want to be leaner, you need to train your body to burn more fat, not just calories. This process can't be rushed, so it is better to choose an activity that feels comfortable. Start with walking rather than running. Walk at a pace you consider "somewhat hard," not difficult. If you are breathing too hard, or your muscles tire quickly, you need to slow down. The "talk test" is an excellent measure of how fast you should go. If you're walking so fast that you can't maintain a conversation or sing a song, just slow it down.

Fat can only be burned "aerobically," that is, when oxygen is available to the muscles. When you first begin to exercise, or when the exercise is too hard, oxygen isn't available to the muscles. Under these conditions, carbohydrates and other fuels supply the energy, not fat. For an activity to be aerobic, it must be performed for at least ten to fifteen minutes.

It's entirely possible that you had a terrible exercise experience at some time in your life. Perhaps a "sadistic" gym teacher made you run laps or do pushups until you just couldn't do anymore. Or you were forced to try and keep up with people who were in better shape than you, until you collapsed.

This old-style whip-you-into-shape approach probably left you feeling like a wimp and swearing off exercise for life. The goal is not to run yourself into the ground as quickly as possible. The goal is to choose an exercise pace that makes you feel good, not bad. If you are worn out after five minutes it doesn't mean you're a wimp. It simply means that you have chosen a pace that is too hard for your body for now.

Your body needs a certain amount of carbohydrate (or sugar) to supply energy during exercise. If you exercise at too high a level for your body, you will burn more sugar than fat and quickly use up your sugar stores. That's when the exercise feels too hard and you feel like quitting. Exercising at a slower pace allows you to save your carbohydrates (sugar) and burn more fat. This makes it possible for you to exercise longer without tiring and ultimately for you to burn more fat and calories.

You may also want to work out at home by following the "Stefanie Powers' Broadway Workout," an exercise video put together with the overweight and newly slim person in mind. It's a "gently gently" step-by-step program, which motivates you to "get up and move" to some of Broadway's all-time hit tunes.

There's someone just like you in this video. There are dieters in their twenties, and a couple of grandmothers; dieters who lost a few pounds, and others who have shed more than forty pounds; women and men; some were already exercise enthusiasts while others were raw beginners. Mother of four Ronda Woodward, 35, has been active for as long as she can remember. She took gymnastics throughout her childhood and, as a teenager, enjoyed cheerleading and waterskiing. She has also taught aerobics and completed a marathon.

Nevertheless, over the years, she has struggled with "the same ten pounds." The Micro Diet helped her lose fifteen pounds after the birth of her last child; exercise has helped her keep it off. In addition to the "Broadway Workout" routines, Ronda alternates running three miles a day with walking five miles a day. Says Ronda, who lives in Park City, Utah, "Exercise makes you feel so good about yourself. It gives you a feeling of well-being and wholeness. I advise people to find an activity that they enjoy doing and capitalize on it."

Conversely, fifty-year-old Dan Kiel, of Sultan, Washington, was a regular couch potato until he lost forty pounds with The Micro Diet. "I was always tired and listless. I had no desire to be physically active, I had too many health problems to worry about." Since losing the weight four years ago, Dan's blood pressure, which was 148/106 is down to 127/78, and his cholesterol reading has dropped from 270 to 160. Says Dan, who now weighs the same as he did the day he graduated from high school, "I use the Stefanie Powers tape three times a week, and I walk a lot. After working out I feel awake and full of energy. In fact, I feel as well as I did back in high school."

Fifty-eight-year-old grandmother of thirteen, Nancy Murray has also lost forty pounds, and is going for another thirty. "If you don't exercise, you're cheating yourself of the full value of The Micro Diet," she says. "If 'life happenings' get me off schedule and I don't exercise, I really notice. My weight stays the same, but my body feels different. Exercise is so energizing and invigorating. I think clearer and always feel one hundred percent better." Exercise for Nancy, of El Cajon, California, means walking at least three times a week, riding a stationary bicycle, and working out to the video. She maintains that, as a society, we spend too much time sitting and driving, and take better care of our cars and pets than we do our own bodies. "Exercise is like getting your own engine charged," she says. When she first started walking for exercise a year ago, she would be tired after the first fifteen minutes. Now she walks over an hour without feeling fatigued. "The more I walk, the farther I want to go. My body pushes me. I've never been as focused and physically active in my life."

Thirty-three-year-old Joanie MacPherson, of San Diego, California, a registered nurse specializing in open-heart surgery, says, "For me, exercise is a stress reliever and motivator in today's fast-paced world. Exercise helps you believe in yourself and lets you have control over your whole being. It has increased my self-confidence tremendously. The key to a sound mind and body is diet and exercise. Because I'm a nurse, I've always known what I need to eat, but I've learned so much from The Micro Diet. I'm much more aware of nutrition and have never felt healthier."

Joanie, who lost ten pounds with The Micro Diet, continues to use the meals as a nutritional supplement. She works out four days a week, alternating between high- and low-impact aerobics, the treadmill, Stairmaster, walking, biking, playing tennis, and swimming.

Like many people, Teresa Zoll, of Medford, Oregon, was very active during her school years but slackened off after entering the workplace, and gained weight. Twenty-five-year-old Teresa lost twenty-five pounds thanks to The Micro Diet, and credits her exercise schedule with helping to keep the weight off.

She began slowly, walking just fifteen minutes a day, and then turned to aerobics. When she couldn't find a class that really suited her, she decided to become an instructor herself. "My energy level is great. Exercise is part of my everyday life. I feel so much better, physically, and mentally."

Karen Forscutt was extremely active as a teenager. Her father managed a roller rink and she could be found there seven days a week. In her twenties she was a jogging and jump-roping enthusiast. In her thirties, she joined a spa where she did aerobics three times a week. Now approaching forty, she prefers to work out to videos in her home in Yadkinville, North Carolina, and play an occasional game of tennis.

With The Micro Diet she got rid of twenty-five pounds in three months and went from a size fourteen to a size six. "I made a conscious effort to exercise. I was never naturally thin, so I had a lot of motivation to maintain my weight and body shape."

## *GET SOCIAL*

One easy way of making exercise fun is to do it with other

people. Join a walking group or start one yourself. Swimming. Cycling. Aerobic dance class. There are many options.

Says Dr. Horton, "It's important to have a variety of activities so that you don't get bored and to choose exercise which can fit into your lifestyle. If you can build exercise into your daily living experience, the chances of long-term success are much better."

Maybe you have looked at someone running or bicycling and wondered how they could endure such discomfort? The answer is that they are not "enduring" anything. As your body becomes used to exercise, or as you lose weight, you will find that you can pick up the pace, move up to a higher level of intensity, and have a great time doing it.

Getting your body in shape is like learning to play a musical instrument. Everything looks difficult before you start, but after you've practiced at a certain level, it becomes easier and you naturally progress to the next level. So, practice taking one step at a time. With time, patience, and action, you'll begin to experience the benefits and wonder why it took you so long to actually get started. You will find that your psychological state gets a real boost. You'll be proud of yourself when you finish your walk or exercise routine—the hormones released by exercise actually make you feel happier.

Go for it, just like four-time Canadian power-lifting champion and Olympic trainer, Bill Gvoich. An author and lecturer, Bill, 42, has worked with the Detroit Red Wings hockey team and professional Canadian teams from a variety of sports. But despite his lifelong commitment to fitness, he accumulated an extra unwanted twenty-five pounds.

January 1, 1992, saw him make a New Year's resolution: To make his body his "science project" using The Micro Diet and a full daily exercise routine. Two months later he had lost the twenty-five pounds and was back in shape. Says Bill, who now runs a wellness program for disabled and elderly patients in St. Petersburg, Florida, "I read all of the literature on The Micro Diet and I was particularly impressed with the balanced nutrition. Combine that with exercise and you've really got something."

Bill started exercising with a five-minute jog. "My knees began to hurt and I could have pushed a little more, but I said 'Hey, that's enough.' Less than two months later I was out for a sixty-three-minute jog. Now I'm able to say 'I've done it! I've researched it. I'm a result of the product.'"

Adds Bill, "For me it wasn't enough to lose weight. I wanted to make sure I lost fat and kept lean body tissue, and increased my strength. I kept a daily diary documenting my food intake—between sixteen hundred and two thousand calories—as well as my jogging, walking, and weight training. Well, I did lose all the fat and kept the muscle. I have abdominals again. Toning is important, too."

Bill is so impressed with his success in combining The Micro Diet with his exercise regimen that he wants to spread the word to other athletes. "It really lends itself to physical activity. It's a great formula for athletic performance. I come from a background of traditional nutrition. I don't believe in popping pills. When I looked at The Micro Diet, I appreciated the fact that this was real food providing all of the nutrients that the body needs without a lot of calories. It is much more than a weight-loss product."

## *# MINUTES TO EXERCISE PER DAY TO BURN UP 2,000 CALORIES A WEEK**

| # Days Exercise Per Week | 3 | 4 | 5 | 6 | 7 |
|---|---|---|---|---|---|
| # Calories Burned Per Day | 667 | 500 | 400 | 333 | 286 |
| Aerobics (heavy) | 74 | 56 | 45 | 37 | 32 |
| Bicycling (10 mph) | 107 | 81 | 65 | 54 | 46 |
| Gardening | 185 | 139 | 111 | 93 | 80 |
| Housework | 148 | 111 | 89 | 74 | 64 |
| Jogging (10 mins. a mile) | 60 | 44 | 35 | 30 | 25 |
| Tennis (singles) | 91 | 69 | 55 | 46 | 89 |
| Walking (20 mins. a mile) | 167 | 125 | 100 | 83 | 72 |

*based on 150-pound person

## *# MINUTES TO EXERCISE PER DAY TO BURN UP 350 CALORIES A WEEK***

| # Days Exercise Per Week | 3 | 4 | 5 | 6 | 7 |
|---|---|---|---|---|---|
| # Calories Burned Per Day | 117 | 88 | 70 | 58 | 50 |
| Aerobics (light) | 26 | 20 | 16 | 13 | 11 |
| Bicycling (6 mph) | 22 | 17 | 13 | 11 | 10 |
| Gardening | 24 | 18 | 15 | 12 | 11 |
| Housework | 20 | 15 | 12 | 10 | 9 |
| Swimming (slow) | 60 | 44 | 35 | 30 | 25 |
| Tennis (doubles) | 16 | 12 | 9 | 8 | 7 |
| Walking (26 mins. a mile) | 26 | 20 | 16 | 13 | 11 |

**based on 200-pound person

Higher Weight (starting):

1. Note that lower intensity activities are chosen, e.g., light instead of heavy aerobics, bicycling at 6 m.p.h., rather than 10 m.p.h., walking instead of jogging, etc.
2. There is a smaller initial goal—to burn 350 calories a week instead of 2,000.
3. Remember, doing a little bit over a long period of time adds up. It's easy and more comfortable to start at this level and gradually step up to the higher level.

## *HOW TO BURN 2,000 CALORIES A WEEK*

Your first course of action is to choose the number of days you wish to exercise: three, four, five, six, or seven. Choose one of the activities listed or, for variety, a combination of them to achieve the required calorie burn. The calculations are based on a 150-pound person.

Seven days a week = 286 calories burned per day:

32 minutes heavy aerobics
46 minutes bicycling (10 mph)
79 minutes gardening
63 minutes housework
25 minutes jogging (10 mins. a mile)
60 minutes walking

Six days a week = 333 calories burned per day:

37 minutes heavy aerobics
54 minutes bicycling (10 mph)
93 minutes gardening
74 minutes housework
30 minutes jogging (10 mins. a mile)
84 minutes walking

Five days a week = 400 calories burned per day:

44 minutes heavy aerobics
64 minutes bicycling (10 mph)
111 minutes gardening
88 minutes housework
35 minutes jogging (10 mins. a mile)
101 minutes walking

Four days a week = 500 calories burned per day:

55 minutes heavy aerobics
80 minutes bicycling (10 mph)
138 minutes gardening
110 minutes housework
44 minutes jogging (10 mins. a mile)
126 minutes walking

Three days a week = 667 calories burned per day:

74 minutes heavy aerobics
107 minutes bicycling (10 mph)
184 minutes gardening
147 minutes housework
59 minutes jogging (10 mins. a mile)
168 minutes walking

## ■ A CASE STUDY

### LAURA KIEL: COMING UNGLUED—FROM THE FRIDGE

Laura Kiel wasn't interested in fast weight loss; she was much more concerned with making sure it stayed off. With a history of yo-yo dieting, Laura made up her mind that it was time to effect permanent change. "I had lost weight lots of times, so I knew I could do that. But every time it would be back within months, sometimes sooner. I developed no skills to help me keep it off. The Micro Diet opened a whole new chapter to my life."

Laura, who originally weighed 267 pounds, lost 107 pounds over a three-and-a-half-year period. She lost thirty pounds and maintained for six months. Then she got rid of twenty-five pounds and maintained that for six months. Her third round of dieting produced a thirty-five-pound loss. She kept at her new weight for ten months before losing seventeen more pounds. Eight months later she is working on her final fifteen pounds.

"I knew I had to take my weight off in that kind of process instead of all at once. I didn't gain the weight in a hurry, so I figured I could take it off in a fairly leisurely manner. I realize that many people prefer faster weight loss, but each weight loss victory gave me renewed confidence that I could move on to the next level. I couldn't handle the thought of losing it all and gaining it all back. I've stayed very mentally healthy the entire time," she says. "Being thin wasn't my main motive when I started The Micro Diet; I was more interested in becoming healthier."

Laura, of Bellevue, Washington, painfully remembers embarrassing moments when she was overweight. "As a nineteen-year-old bride-to-be I was in a shop looking for my wedding dress. After attempting to get into dress after dress the clerk turned to me and said, 'You're just thick through the middle.' I was crushed and I left in tears. Years later I ran into my aunt while shopping and she hadn't seen me in a long time. Her first comment was, 'Oh, You're pregnant again?' I wasn't pregnant, and my daughter was two years old at the time."

In those days, Laura would—even after dinner—spend the evening "glued to the refrigerator." Often she would get out of bed in the middle of the night to eat a sandwich. She began The Micro Diet by making a five-day commitment. "My patient and loving

Advisor encouraged me to give it five days. I enjoyed the products I lost weight and, for the first time, I could see the possibility of successfully managing my weight. Those five days changed my life. Food is no longer the controlling force in my life. Yes, I love food and because of The Micro Diet I am learning the necessary skills to become slim, stay slim, and still love food. I have a whole new outlook on life. I feel like someone has put me in a photocopier and reduced me in half."

At a recent family reunion her relatives, says Laura, "were shocked to see that I hadn't regained my weight. It's funny, though, because many people can't remember what I used to look like and I have to show them a picture to make them appreciate how much weight I have lost. My mother saw a 'before' photo of me the other day and couldn't believe it. She had simply forgotten what I looked like at that weight."

# 13

# RE-EDUCATING YOUR PALATE

MANY PEOPLE DO HAVE A natural tendency to gain weight easily. But there is also no avoiding the fact that overeating is the major cause of obesity. A person who only needs 1,200 calories of food a day is overeating on 1,500 calories, even though 1,500 calories is relatively low compared with the average person's energy needs.

If you fall into this category, it is undoubtedly unfair; but once you have lost your excess fat, having failed so many times before, you can switch your priority to maintaining your new trimmer physique. Most loser-friendly dieters continue using Micro meals to replace one or two meals a day or when it is a convenient part of their lifestyle.

Take Sal Serio of Port St. Lucie, Florida, for example. He has learned how to incorporate Micro meals into his everyday lifestyle as a way of maintaining his weight. It obviously works for him, as Sal lost ninety-two pounds in 1987, and has kept it off. Says Sal, "I have learned to eat whatever I want at the appropriate time. For instance, Memorial Day is coming up. On the weekend I will eat whatever I please and, afterward, I will use The Micro Diet 'sole source' for a few days, or have two Micro meals a day plus other food for three days. I never deprive myself, so I never feel like I'm on a diet.

"The Micro Diet is a way of life for me. It's not a diet. It's food everybody needs. Why wouldn't you want to put something so nutritious into your body every day? I have a shake for breakfast and I simply don't feel hungry until much later in the day."

Sal says that he had had a weight problem for as long as he could remember—"I think I was born two hundred fifty pounds"—and got to the point where he didn't want to leave the house. He was constantly trying different ways to lose weight. "Every Monday I would start a diet and every Thursday, Friday, and Saturday I would blow it. I would crave food and go on an eating binge. It seems to me that many of us fill ourselves up with empty calories—junk food. We don't get the nutrition we need and then we're hungry again. What made The Micro Diet so different from other plans was that it eliminated those cravings, and seeing the weight come off so quickly gave me the incentive to stay with the program. I lost nineteen pounds in the first fourteen days and was feeling better than at any time in my life. That got me excited."

Sal knows, too, that it is important to make a determined effort to shed those excess pounds. "You have got to make a total commitment. I like to say that you *get rid of* weight and not lose weight. When you get rid of something you never want it back; when you lose something you normally want to find it again. I got rid of my weight and I'm positive I will never find it again. The Micro Diet taught me to be in control of my life. I don't step on scales any more. I now have a lot of muscle and can easily knock out a hundred push-ups" but, he hastily adds, "I had to work up to that point."

Says Lynne Wright, 44, of Bakersfield, California, who dropped thirty-one pounds in ten weeks and regained a shapely 37–26–36 figure, "This isn't a 'can't' diet, it's a positive 'can' diet. I've spent hundreds of dollars and countless hours of anxiety trying to lose weight, but the morning I stepped on the bathroom scales and realized I had become heavier than the day I'd delivered twins twenty-three years earlier, I was devastated.

"Being overweight is a very personal thing. Losing twenty pounds can be as important to one person as losing fifty or one hundred pounds is to someone else. This makes it a very emotional issue as well as a health problem. One's self-image is often tied to that reflection in the mirror. When that reflection no longer fits our 'good image' we can be merciless in berating the physical person we have become. Enter the yo-yo syndrome and the cycle of defeat. The Micro Diet is a tool not only to lose weight but to maintain a healthy weight. I no longer think of The Micro Diet as a diet. It is simply the new and healthy way to live and eat.

In our busy daily life or travels, it enables me to always have a well-balanced meal at hand."

It is extremely important to bear in mind that long-term weight maintenance entails reducing food intake permanently. If you go back to eating the same amount of food that you did when you were overweight, the fat is definitely going to come piling back on! For every two pounds of weight lost, the newly slim person needs to consume sixteen to twenty calories less. So, if the dieter has lost forty-four pounds, to maintain that weight loss, he or she must eat 300 to 400 calories a day less than before losing the weight.

The prime aim of this section of the book is to make you aware of changes you can make in your everyday eating habits to help you keep the weight off.

There is only so much information that can be effectively shared through the medium of a book. I strongly recommend, therefore, that you obtain a copy of The Micro Diet's *Choices* program. It's a unique, interactive compendium of useful information and exercises—including audio tapes, booklets, flash cards, and charts—designed to ensure that you never become overweight again.

## *SO WHY DO YOU EAT?*

Do you eat to live or live to eat? Some people view food emotionally. They eat for all sorts of reasons other than simple hunger: boredom, worry, stress, habit, impulse. We eat for "mind" reasons as well as "body" reasons.

It is important to view food in its proper perspective: to be enjoyed, relished, something absolutely necessary, of course, but not something to dominate our thoughts or be an emotional crunch. Think carefully about these questions and answer them honestly and fully:

### Do you ever eat to reward yourself?

You worked hard today, coped especially well with the children, helped a friend, so you ate something special.

### Do you always finish everything on your plate?

It is immoral to waste food, right? Wrong! Scandalous when there are starving children in the Third World, right? Wrong! It is illogical to overburden your body with more than you need, and the starving children would be better off with a donation to a suitable charity.

**Do you eat absentmindedly?**

Do you pick at leftovers while talking? Munch snacks while watching TV? One of the best examples of "mindless calories" is when you go to the movies. You buy a box of popcorn or chocolate. The first two mouthfuls are delicious. Then you go on "automatic pilot." Your hand keeps dipping into the box and finding its own way toward your mouth. The next thing you know is that there are none left and you never even noticed you were eating them. Pure mindless calories!

**Do you eat because you're bored?**

There's not much to do. You're alone. So you make yourself something to eat. Everybody does it but some of us do it a lot too often.

**Do you eat when you're worried?**

Everybody gets tense and anxious. Nervous under pressure. So you eat. You're a little unsure of yourself at a social occasion. So you eat. It's something to do with your hands. Funny, because that's exactly what smokers say. Eating because you are worried may well seem a "natural reaction" to you but it is not going to make the problem go away. In fact, you may well end up with an additional problem: being overweight.

Kristy Tidwell, of Fort Bragg, California, confesses that she was always heavy but blames a combination of kicking the nicotine habit and emotional stress for her excessive weight gain.

"In November of 1988 my weight problem started accelerating. I quit smoking (with no regrets!) and immediately started substituting food for cigarettes," she says. "Just about the time I was beginning to get control of my food, my mother died suddenly. I was devastated and heartsick. I again turned to food for consolation and ballooned to two hundred and ninety pounds. My all-time high. I was frantic and desperate for help. I had the feeling that if I went over three hundred pounds I would be lost forever.

"Then one evening I turned on the television and there was a weight-loss show. It has been a love affair with The Micro Diet ever since. I've lost one hundred and eight pounds. For the first time in my life I truly like myself. I have loads of energy and a whole new positive outlook on life."

**Do you eat because it is lunchtime?**

Many people eat simply because of the time of day. It's 8:00 A.M., so breakfast is required. At 1:00 P.M. it is time to take a break from work and go for lunch. Or it is 6:00 P.M. and the family is all at home for dinner. You might not be hungry, but the eating routine has to be kept.

**Do you eat because it is nighttime?**

You have a late supper (as a kind of sleeping pill), or you find yourself waking up in the night and raiding the refrigerator. Could this be because you don't have three balanced meals a day?

Suzanne de Rham describes herself as a "revolving eater." Teenage daughter, Cathy, would arrive home "on empty" after band practice at 4:30 P.M. Suzanne herself would be hungry again and eat between 6:00 P.M. and 8:00 P.M. Husband Fred could arrive home at any time between 8:00 P.M. and 2:00 A.M.—usually unfed and starving. Suzanne would then handle inventory for their business between 2:00 A.M. and 4:00 A.M. and stop at Denny's on the way home or raid the refrigerator, "usually something fast and fattening."

Says Suzanne, "I would eat at all of these times, and with my husband and daughter to be 'friendly.' "

The net result was that Suzanne gained an extra twenty-two unwanted pounds. As a former Miss Louisville and first runner-up in the Miss Kentucky pageant those twenty-two pounds weighed very heavily on her mind. Yet, in little over a month, thanks to The Micro Diet, she was back to the weight and shape she had boasted twenty-nine years earlier when she held those beauty queen titles. Today, five years later, Suzanne, of Ormond Beach, Florida, has maintained her weight loss and can still slip into the bathing suit she wore back in 1958.

How does she do it? "The Micro Diet is my health insurance policy. I find myself eating Micro meals for at least one meal a day, almost always two meals, sometimes three meals and once in a while, four meals. This constitutes my nutritional base. The Micro Diet is my 'basic food group.' " Adds Suzanne, "I was exceedingly pleased when I was able to get into the wedding dress I had worn at thirty-five years of age; but I'm ecstatic to be able to slip into that bathing suit thirty-three years later without ripping a single brittle thread. I have one vital piece of advice for everyone trying to maintain their weight: Buy a good quality leather belt when you reach your ideal weight. Mark the notch on the back of the belt, wear the belt regularly, and never move the buckle to another notch. If the belt gets snug, go back on The Micro Diet as your sole source of nutrition for a day or two and drink lots of water. I can proudly show my 'one-notch,' well-worn belt to everyone and demonstrate that my size has stayed very, very constant."

**Do you eat to be polite?**

You're attending a business lunch and don't feel you should risk abusing your host's hospitality? Your friend wants you to sample the cake she has just baked? You don't have to do it! If you explain that you have to watch your weight they will understand.

**Do you eat because you love to cook?**

You're a gastronomic overeater! The entire ceremony of food preparation appeals to you. You may not sit down to a huge meal because you've eaten so much while cooking. A high percentage of people in this category are actually male.

These are just a few reasons why we eat and overeat. Some of them are physical, but many were really feeding your mind. It's your body, however, that picked up the extra calories. Do you know how big your stomach is? Make a fist and look at it. That's how little food it takes to fill your stomach. If you feel that you, too, may eat for reasons other than nutrition, answer just a few more questions and then we can start to deal with the issue. Think back to when you first noticeably put on weight. What was your age? Your financial situation? How were your relationships—with your parents, your friends, the opposite sex?

**What did your answers to the above questions tell you about yourself?**

They probably brought home to you how often you eat for reasons quite unconnected with being hungry. The chances are that some of your eating is really a reflex action. Unthinking. If you need to keep your weight under control, you can't afford to indulge in calories you don't fully enjoy.

Here's a project that's fun and will be a revelation. At the next convenient weekend make a favorite meal. Try and ensure that it includes a really tasty meat or fish dish and your favorite vegetables, plus a good choice of fresh fruit. Include a luscious dessert. Now spread it all on the table before you start. Pick up the plate, look carefully at each piece of food. Take up a piece on your fork. Smell it. Savor it. Now chew it carefully and concentrate on the taste and texture. Did you know that the taste of food is different depending on whether it touches the front or back of your tongue?

Now do the same for every different type of food on your plate. Notice which you liked most. Now start again, eating slowly, and relishing each item. Stop to consider how hungry you are. Continue and stop frequently to ask yourself the same question, "Am I still hungry?" When you have reached the point that you can sense that you're no longer hungry, simply stop eating.

Perhaps for the first time in a long while you will have really concentrated on your food, appreciated it, sensed its effect. It should have been a sensually pleasurable experience rather than the rushed grab we so often make our eating occasions. And what do you do with any food left when you have stopped? Throw it away. After you've done that, notice how you felt about the meal and about throwing the leftovers away.

## *HIDDEN CALORIES*

I don't believe in endless calorie counting, but that doesn't mean you can ignore the calories or the caloric value of certain foods. If you know the type of food to treat with great caution, you do not have to bother counting calories in the sort of food that, in practice, you won't overeat.

So the concept of "hidden calories" is useful. They are the foods that are surprisingly caloric. Here are just a few of those surprises!

SALAD DRESSING (250 calories extra)

Salads can be unlimited, right? Yes—but salad dressing certainly can't. Just two ounces casually poured over the salad is often 250 calories.

SOUR CREAM (60 calories extra)

A baked potato is an ideal food. The sour cream ladled on it probably costs at least sixty calories.

BRAN MUFFINS (336 calories extra)

A mid-morning break with three bran muffins. The muffins alone cost 336 calories—that's equivalent to one hour of brisk walking. Worth it? The choice is yours.

GRILLED FISH WITH BUTTER (110 calories extra)

The grilled fish was a great decision—but the half ounce of butter added more than 100 casual, hidden calories.

A NONFAT CHOCOLATE BAR (320 calories)

Two ounces of chocolate will give you a quick energy fix, but an hour later it leaves you feeling hungry. It's all too easy to eat a bar of chocolate, for example, while driving the car. Three hundred and twenty mindless calories!

A SLICE OF HOT APPLE PIE (250 calories)

Some snacks are just loaded with hidden calories.

PEANUT BUTTER (35 calories)

Just one teaspoon is thirty-five calories, so think again before having a taste or liberally spreading on bread.

QUICHE (585 calories)

What about this one? We think of a slice of quiche as a healthy, nourishing food. But an average slice of five ounces/150g costs 585 calories. Beware!

AVOCADO (235 calories)

Just half an appetizing avocado!

Let's be clear. I'm not saying that you can't have any of the above. I am saying you shouldn't mislead yourself by ignoring the "hidden calories." Being aware of these hidden calories in the "extras" is half the battle. For instance, think back to the last time you went to a cafeteria. Do you know what's often displayed first, as you start sliding your tray down the counter? Desserts, cream cakes, ice cream. That's because restaurateurs know that when you're hungry you won't be able to resist helping yourself to precisely that type of food.

Here is a suggestion for when you are next in a cafeteria. Buy the main course first, chicken or fish, for example. Then, when you've eaten that, ask yourself, "Do I really want dessert?" You'll notice a big difference in your attitude. First, you have to consider whether you want to be bothered with standing in line all over again. Second, you are now questioning whether you really want dessert, after you have already begun to feel full. So now if you do want the dessert you are making a conscious decision—not an unthinking grab for food at the very moment you are likely to make the worst choices, i.e., when you are hungry!

## *THE EASY CHANGES*

Preparing food becomes, after a time, a matter of habit. Yet it's quite possible to eliminate an amazing number of calories by really simple changes. The point about these changes is that, individually, they don't seem to amount to much, even over the course of a month. Yet, over a year, each one can make a real impact, and several changes together will accumulate to a dramatic effect.

Here is a list of some easy changes you can make. Your body is not like an adding (or subtracting) machine, so you can't assume that just because you cut out, for example, four teaspoonfuls of sugar a day, you will automatically lose twelve pounds a year. The relationship, in practice, between calories and weight loss is not that simple, but the list indicates the exciting potential.

I hope more examples are superfluous. There is no food that is truly "off limits." But by making sensible substitutes, you can effect savings that over the course of a year have an impressive impact. Reread the list and think about it.

What did you do? You:

1. Cut out sugar in tea and coffee. It really can be done in a couple of weeks. You'll hate the taste the first day. Persevere and, by the end of the second week, you'll probably hate the taste of sugar.
2. You ate more chicken, fish, and lean red meat and less high fat, processed, and highly marbled cuts.
3. You used low-calorie mixers, club soda, and diet soft drinks.
4. You broiled your food instead of frying it.
5. You used skimmed milk.
6. You used low-calorie margarine and spread the jam just enough to taste.
7. You used broth-based soup, not cream soup.

## THE EASY CHANGES

| What You May Do Now | What You Could Do | Calories It Would Save Each Time | Calories It Would Save in a Year | How Many Lbs. Less It Would Be |
|---|---|---|---|---|
| 2 t of powdered coffee creamer per cup of coffee (say 4 cups a day) | Stop adding creamer. Drink black. | 20 cal. per cup, i.e., 80 cal. per day | 29,200 | 8½ lbs. |
| You use 5 oz. whole milk on your cereal (3 times a week). 75 calories | Use 5 oz. skimmed or nonfat milk. 42 calories | 100 calories | 5,148 | 1½ lbs. |
| You have 2 slices of toast & jam using 2 tsp. butter and 1 T jam (twice a week). 280 calories | Have 2 slices of toast & jam using 2 t diet margarine and 1 T low-sugar jam. 200 calories | 160 calories | 8,320 | 2⅓ lbs. |
| Quarter Pounder from fast food restaurant (twice a week). 848 calories | Turkey sandwich 3 oz. turkey with mustard & no mayo from local deli (twice a week). 600 calories | 248 calories | 12,896 | 3½ lbs. |
| Tuna salad sandwich made with 3 oz. tuna, oil packed, with 1 T mayo & pickle relish served on Pita (once a week). 437 calories | Tuna salad sandwich made with 2 oz. water-packed tuna, ½ cup chopped carrots, celery, cauliflower, ½ T light mayo served on Pita (once a week). 300 calories | 137 calories | 7,124 | 2 lbs. |

## THE EASY CHANGES

| What You May Do Now | What You Could Do | Calories It Would Save Each Time | Calories It Would Save in a Year | How Many Lbs. Less It Would Be |
|---|---|---|---|---|
| You have a bowl of cream soup (tomato, clam chowder, etc.). 6 oz./120 calories | Choose a bowl of broth-based soup (vegetable, minestrone, etc.). 6 oz./80 calories | 40 calories | 2,080 | ½ lb. |
| 5- 4 oz. glasses of wine a week | Drink only 2- 4 oz. glasses of wine a week | 360 cal. per week | 18,720 | 5⅓ lbs. |
| Snack on 16 Wheat Thins & 1 oz. cheddar cheese (3 times a week) | Switch to 2 Rye Krisp crackers & 1 oz. mozzarella cheese (3 times a week). 122 calories | 138 cal. per snack<br>414 cal. per week | 21,528 | 6 lbs. |
| 1 small package Doritos corn chips (once a week) | Same amount of chips made by baking plain corn tortillas in 400° oven. | 73 calories | 3,796 | 1 lb. |
| 2 T blue cheese salad dressing (3 times a week). 150 calories. | 2 T low-calorie Italian dressing (3 times a week). 40 calories. | 330 calories | 17,160 | 5 lbs. |
| 6 oz. chicken, fried with skin (once a week). 550 calories. | 6 oz. chicken, broiled without skin (once a week). 400 calories. | 150 calories | 7,880 | 2 lbs. |

## THE EASY CHANGES

| What You May Do Now | What You Could Do | Calories It Would Save Each Time | Calories It Would Save in a Year | How Many Lbs. Less It Would Be |
|---|---|---|---|---|
| Use 2 Tbs of cooking oil in chicken vegetable stir-fry | Use non-stick pan & cut oil to ¾ Tbs. (add water or chicken broth if necessary) | 158 cal. per spoon | 16,430 | 5 lbs. |
| Order 10 oz. prime rib at restaurant (twice a month). 1000 calories. | Order 2 pieces chicken, batter dipped & fried with skin—all the better when you find broiled without skin (twice a week). 578 calories. | 422 calories | 21,944 | 6 lbs. |
| You have 6 oz. breaded, deep-fat fried fish & french fries. 640 calories. | You have 6 oz. char-broiled fish & medium baked potato with 1 Tbs. sour cream. 326 calories. | 314 calories | 16,328 | 4½ lbs. |
| You have apple pie & ½ cup ice cream. 282 cal. + 150 cal. 432 calories. | You have ½ piece apple pie & ¼ cup ice cream. 141 cal. + 75 cal. 216 cal. | 216 calories | 11,232 | 3 lbs. |
| 1 spoon of sugar per cup of tea or coffee (say 4 cups a day) | Use non-calorie sweetener | 15 calories per tsp., 60 cal. per day | 21,900 | 6¼ lbs. |

## THE EASY CHANGES

| What You May Do Now | What You Could Do | Calories It Would Save Each Time | Calories It Would Save in a Year | How Many Lbs. Less It Would Be |
|---|---|---|---|---|
| Snack 1 packet (2 oz.) peanuts while watching TV (twice a week). | Only eat at the table, therefore NO TV snacks. | 324 cal. per packet, 648 cal. per week | 33,700 | 10 lbs. |
| Drink gin & tonic (4 drinks a week). | Switch to low-calorie tonic. | 40 cal. per drink 160 cal. per week | 8,320 | 2½ lbs. |
| 4 fried eggs in fat (once a week). | Fry in non-stick pan without fat or oil. | 20 cal. per egg 80 cal. per week | 4,160 | 1¼ lb. |
| You use mayonnaise for Prawn Cocktail. | You mix ⅓ mayonnaise with ⅔ yogurt. | 67 cal. per portion | varies | varies |
| You make a Beef Stroganoff using 5 oz. sour cream. | You use 3 oz. natural yogurt. | 65 cal. per portion | varies | varies |
| You make tomato salad using vinaigrette dressing. | You use lemon juice instead. | 145 cal. average per person per serving | varies | varies |

Salad dressings use a high proportion of oil which is very, very caloric. Use yogurt or lemon juice. The true taste of the salad is better preserved.

8. You substituted plain yogurt for cream and mayonnaise.
9. You used lemon juice instead of vinaigrette or oil dressing.

None of the above changes were exactly traumatic, were they? You are still eating the same kinds of foods, but the accumulative effect over the course of a year could be a saving of tens of thousands of calories! You've potentially saved pounds of fat compared with the result of continuing the old habits. See how a few cooking changes can help you maintain your weight? See how much margin for error you have by making the easy changes? And remember that as a "safety net" you always have the opportunity to go back on The Micro Diet "sole source" for a day or two.

# 14

# CHANGING YOUR HABITS

HABITS—GOOD AND BAD—are the ways you have learned to do things. The "learning" is the end result of constant repetition of the way you respond to a common situation. Habits are not something we often consciously form, but to change them does require conscious effort. It also requires patience and practice. The reason you were overeating—compared with your personal metabolic needs—was probably because you just didn't realize that your body needed fewer calories and because you were operating on "automatic pilot." Your job is to "program" that automatic pilot with a different set of instructions.

## *RECOGNIZING THE PROBLEM*

The best possible way to be conscious of your current habits is quite simply to take two pieces of paper. On one piece of paper write down everything that you eat tomorrow. "Everything" means exactly that: meals, snacks, tasting food which you are cooking, tidbits, and don't forget milk and sugar in tea or coffee.

You must also record what you were doing at the time—standing by the refrigerator, watching TV, reading, sitting at the table. Then do the same for the next day. It really should not take more than five minutes. What it will do is surprise you. You will probably be staggered at the number of occasions you eat other than sitting at your table. It's a safe bet that you also find yourself eating for reasons other than hunger. You may be surprised, too, when you remember your mood while you were eating. Were you fed up, worried, bored? That's significant, isn't it?

## *TAKE IT EASY*

Just relax, mentally, and physically. Try not to get uptight about being on a diet. Don't get bent out of shape because someone else is losing weight faster than you are. Remember, we are all unique individuals. If you're bored, anxious, frustrated, or just plain mad at the world, go for a walk. Just don't turn to food.

## *DEVELOP A "FAT-FREE" HOME*

Does your home resemble a 7-11 store? No matter where you turn can you conveniently lay your hands on something edible and loaded with calories? Clear it out and make a fresh start. Turn your home into a safe house. Try and make it a "fat-free" home.

In the past you have probably rationalized the need for plentiful bags of potato chips and keeping the cookie jar well-stocked on the grounds that the kids or your spouse aren't dieting and they need something to snack on, or you need something to offer any friend who might drop by. Well, they might not need to lose weight today, but they certainly need to eat healthier. So encourage them to support you in your efforts by eliminating those items from the pantry—especially as it's for their own good, as well.

## *WHEN YOU SHOP, USE A LIST AND STICK TO IT. SHOP AS SOON AS POSSIBLE AFTER A MEAL*

Next time you go shopping, plan ahead. Decide what you *do* need and what you really don't need. People make more sensible food choices and purchase less caloric food when they are not hungry.

Please don't just acknowledge this advice, practice it. Make your next shopping trip after you've just eaten, and you'll be amazed at the difference. Always use a shopping list and make sure you only purchase items on the list. Only take enough money with you to cover the cost of the essentials.

## *ALWAYS HAVE THREE MEALS A DAY*

To keep your body satisfied, it is important to eat regularly. Breakfast should not be skipped, but, of course, many of us feel we simply "can't face anything" first thing in the morning or we "just don't have time." A Micro meal is the ideal solution. In one meal, in one minute, you enjoy at least one-third of your day's nutritional requirements. What a great start to the day! Lunch and dinner also have their part to play because, by taking proper nourishment at regular mealtimes, you may dispel the urge to snack between meals.

"I don't skip meals and don't allow myself to get too hungry," says Norma Gilman, of Central Point, Oregon. "I eat to fuel my body, instead of just for the pleasure of eating. In fact, the real pleasure I get from meals today is more from whom I share the meal with rather than what I eat. The convenience of the Micro meals makes it real easy to ensure I have three meals a day. I have at least one Micro meal a day."

Norma lost sixty pounds with The Micro Diet and has maintained her goal weight of 125 pounds for more than two-and-a-half years. "I have lost weight many times over the past thirty years only to steadily gain it back. I was skeptical when I was introduced to The Micro Diet, but after a short time I felt so much better and had so much more energy. It opened the door to a whole new lifestyle for me and enabled me to make a commitment to changing my attitudes and habits. I know I can keep my weight off, but I realize I have to stay on top of it, or I will gain it back."

## *DRINK BEFORE YOU EAT*

When you're preparing dinner, or as soon as you arrive at a restaurant, fill up your tank with water. A nice, cold glass (or more) of sparkling water is refreshing and will keep you from eating so much. Alternatively, have a pitcher of iced tea or other non-caloric drink always at hand.

## *ALWAYS EAT SITTING DOWN AND ALWAYS EAT IN A SPECIFIC PLACE!*

Eating should be something you concentrate on and thoroughly enjoy. My philosophy is that food is great, and eating is one of life's major pleasures. But be a gourmet, not a glutton. People who really love food savor its flavor. You don't have to eat ten ounces of steak to get the taste of steak; six ounces eaten slowly with relish, will taste just as good. If you ever go to a five-star restaurant in France you'll discover two things: The food is exquisite, and the helpings are much smaller than would be served in the U.S. They are gourmets, not gluttons.

The same is true of the Japanese. They eat many courses but each one is a small delicacy. You feast, but you don't feel full. It's a relief to get up from the table and not feel stuffed. Instead, you feel good. The British Royal Family is probably involved in more social eating with more rich food at more lavish banquets than anyone. They eat some of each dish, quite deliberately leaving some of the food so that they are ready for the next course. This way everything can be tasted and enjoyed.

So, if you respect food you will make eating an occasion. You can't concentrate on the taste if you are reading, or watching TV, or doing a crossword. You have no appreciation of how much you eat, or its quality. The same is true about eating standing up. Grabbing something to eat as you walk past the fridge is not respecting food.

If you sit down in one place you will learn to feel the effect of food, learn to eat for taste and not out of boredom. You will also be in a position to sense when you no longer feel hungry. If you mindlessly help yourself to handfuls of peanuts, potato chips, or chocolate while watching TV, you have no chance of registering whether you're hungry or not. Eat in one place. Eat sitting down and concentrate ONLY on eating. Avoid "mindless calories."

## *PRACTICE LEAVING SOMETHING ON YOUR PLATE*

Now, this will be a little harder to swallow! At the beginning of the program, please make a conscious decision to leave something on your plate. There are really good reasons for this. We are trained to eat too much. We start with a natural instinct to stop eating when we are no longer hungry, but this instinct is suppressed. A baby that is breast-fed will eat as much as it needs. Like an animal in the wild, it instinctively stops eating when it is satisfied. When the baby is switched to a bottle, the mother can now see if anything is left, and the reaction of most mothers is to encourage the baby to finish it up, even though if left alone the child would have stopped feeding. Statistically, bottle-fed babies are heavier than breast-fed babies.

So begins the habit of finishing up everything on the plate, the "waste not, want not" adage. When you leave something on your plate, you are saying two things to your subconscious. First, you are saying that you have control, you do not need to eat just because it's there. Second, and of far greater importance, it reduces your emotional and psychological dependence on food. The first time you deliberately leave something you may feel guilty. But do it. Do it at each evening meal for a week and you'll discover a new feeling. You'll no longer feel uneasy at leaving food, you'll feel in control. The beneficial effect on your subconscious attitude to food will be immense.

Don't pass this advice over as a fad piece of psychology—it really works. Also, you should use a small plate to make portions appear larger. And leave the table as soon as you can. This will remove the temptation to pick at what you have left while slower eaters are still dining. It's not rude. It's your health that's at stake.

## *EAT SLOWLY*

Many overweight people "inhale" their food. It's almost as if a vacuum cleaner had been held over their plate. If this is you, make a conscious effort to eat slowly and you will find that it may take as few as twelve bites of food to satisfy your hunger. Try it and observe how you feel. You'll find that the desire to continue eating after the first dozen mouthfuls is mostly for taste, or for social reasons. Alternatively, don't hold an eating utensil in your hand while you have food in your mouth or, instead, try eating with the "wrong" hand. That will slow you down.

All this is part of the general encouragement to listen to your body. If you are aware of it, and in tune with it, you'll gradually get back to the condition you were born with, the ability to eat what you really need, when you really need it.

It can actually take from twenty to forty-five minutes after you start eating before you lose the feeling of hunger, no matter how much food you eat. So spend a full twenty minutes eating your meals—even the lightest meal.

## *AFTER DINNER*

Put the kitchen out of bounds. Try to avoid going anywhere near the refrigerator. It's a good idea to take a pitcher of water into the room where you are going to spend the rest of the evening and drink to your heart's content.

After dinner was the danger time for Bob Goldberg, a warehouse manager and driver who lives in Yorktown Heights, New York. Says Bob, "My wife used to call me a couch potato. I would come home from work, plop down on the couch, and fall asleep watching TV. Then I would be called for dinner. After dinner is when my problem really began. Out came the pretzels, chips, cashews, M & M's. You name it, I ate it. Everyone used to look at me as an old man with a beer belly, even though I was only thirty-seven and didn't drink beer. I just loved to eat."

After losing forty-seven pounds in two-and-a-half months, Bob says, "Everything has changed. I eat right and am able to play with my three kids instead of sleeping on the couch. While watching TV, I exercise, making sure I don't fall back into my old lazy routine. Best of all, after I exercise I feel better, stronger, and have no desire to eat. Everyone sees the new me. They call me 'Slim' at work and I glow with pride. There's not a day goes by that someone I know doesn't remark about how great I look."

Bob has maintained his weight loss for over a year through following better eating habits, and, he says, "because I am very determined to stay thin. I know it's up to me. You can keep the weight off if you really want to."

## *CUT DOWN ON THE SUGAR*

Reducing one's sugar intake is certainly very common advice, and here's why. Sugar has no other nutritional value but calories. It is just "empty calories," absolutely valueless for anything but sweetening and energy.

You can learn to hate it in tea or coffee. Ask anyone who has given it up. If they accidently drink a cup that has been sweetened they feel that it tastes awful. (I know that from personal experience.) By far the best way is to cut down by half for a week, then half again for another week, and by the end of the third week eliminate it altogether. You really can do it. While it is comparatively easy to eliminate sugar from your tea and coffee (and thereby potentially save over 24,000 calories a year), reducing sugar in other ways requires some vigilance. Reading labels on cans and bottles is instructive. An easy way to cut out totally unnecessary calories is never to buy canned fruit in syrup.

## *MAKE YOUR NATURAL LAZINESS WORK FOR YOU*

It is obvious that you can't eat what is not available. I know of dieters who keep no chocolates or candy in the house at all. If they want them they have to go out to the store. So they ask themselves the key question, "I can have it if I want it, but do I really want it?" Mostly they don't.

On a more everyday basis, if you are making toast, put one slice in the toaster at a time. If you make a stack of toast at one time, you'll eat it. If you have to go to the bother of making it one slice at a time you'll definitely eat less. Another absolute rule should be to keep serving dishes away from the table. You won't have the same temptation to have further helpings. In the same way you should dispose of all leftovers. If it's useable at another meal put it in a container and away in the fridge or, even better, the freezer. If it is not, throw it out immediately.

Remember, you can have ANYTHING just as long as you really want it. When you have chocolate have *a* chocolate. Take one or two out of the box then put the box out of sight. Nibble the chocolate, concentrate upon it, and savor it. If you leave an open box in front of you it's amazing how fast it disappears without you even being aware. Mindless calories.

## *WATCH OTHER PEOPLE EAT*

Some people eat very quickly. They don't stop between mouthfuls and they chew only a short time. They start the next course as soon as the previous one is finished. They eat everything on their plate indiscriminately. They attack every meal as if it were their last meal.

Others eat slowly. They put their knife and fork down between mouthfuls. They chew thoroughly. They cut up their food into small pieces and, as a result, it looks substantial on their plate. They have no hesitation in stopping eating when they don't feel hungry. They will leave food on their plates. They realize that if they don't "waste it" they will only "waist it."

## *EAT JUST A LITTLE BIT LESS*

If I can register one fact throughout the loser-friendly program, it is that maintaining an attractive figure and a healthy body is the result of making several small changes. By far the easiest is "eat just a little bit less."

If you burn up 2,100 calories a day (the average woman probably does) and you eat just 5% less (that's 1/20th less of everything), you take in 105 fewer calories a day. You won't notice the difference that day, either in the amount of food or in your weight. Nor will you notice the difference at the end of the week. You probably won't notice much difference at the end of the month, either. But over the course of a year you could save ten pounds.

Research shows just how crucial it is for the person who has lost weight to permanently reduce his or her calorie intake. Professor Jequier at Switzerland's University of Lausanne, for instance, has shown that the metabolic rate of people who have lost forty pounds drops by at least 320 calories a day. On average, you need to reduce your daily calorie intake by about eight calories for every pound of weight you have lost. No wonder so many people put the weight back on. The hard truth is that you do need to cut your calorie intake permanently compared with your calorie (food) intake before you lost your weight.

## *ENLIST A FRIEND*

Family and friends can be the best support system of all. Here are some suggestions you will like. Have someone else do the grocery shopping for you and buy only the things you put on the list. Have someone help you cook food for the following week and freeze it. Have someone else heat it up at mealtime. Whenever possible, don't eat alone, and have your family or guests clean up after meals so you can stay away from extra food.

If you feel you need help, call your Micro Diet Advisor. He or she is your friend. They won't come and do the washing up for you, but they will be supportive of your efforts. Losing weight can be a social activity, which is why meetings are held all over the country. Why not attend such a meeting and team up with a buddy who is also losing weight? You can help each other.

## *COOKING*

One of my colleagues recently talked to a friend who had a weight problem. She was cooking. They were discussing the idea of recording everything she ate for a day because she claimed she ate "very little." The next day she handed over the sheet. She had quite forgotten the fact that she had tasted three different foods at precisely the time the diary was being discussed. If you really have to taste, use a small teaspoon.

I've read of one psychologist who handles patients who just aren't aware that they're eating by recommending that they wear a surgical mask while cooking. He says that it's very effective and that they can discard it after a week!

## *PREPARING FOOD*

How often have you put out "munchies" before a party—potato chips, peanuts, dips, snacks—and found you'd eaten half a plate just by picking each time you walked past? So "hide" them until the last minute. Equally, after the party, put leftovers away immediately.

## *EATING OUT*

It's a simple statement to make but necessary all the same: Avoid going to the "Hungry Heifer's All You Can Eat for $4.95" buffet. It puts too much temptation in your way. When dining in a restaurant, order small portions, if available. Ask for low-cal margarine instead of butter. Order soup or an appetizer instead of the main meal. Better still, decide what you are going to eat before you get to the restaurant (e.g., fresh fish of the day, broiled, no butter). That way you won't have to open the menu and be tempted by those mouth-watering descriptions. If you're with a like-minded companion ask for any freebies to be removed from the table, or keep them at arm's length. Don't be embarrassed about eating half of your dinner and taking the rest home in a doggie bag.

At a party, most of us tend to be a little shy. Eating something can be a way of occupying our hands. Reduce the temptation by deliberately standing away from the snack table. Go through the buffet line without a plate, then have a low-cal drink and, while sipping the drink, decide which items you really do want to have before reapproaching the buffet table. Alternatively, use just a small plate. If you enjoy drinking alcohol why not make every other drink a low-cal drink? You are still drinking, but not so much and no one will notice. Don't forget, alcohol has no nutritional value. It just provides extra calories.

Stanley Schmiedecke, at 6-foot, 9-inches and 380 pounds, was a veritable bear of a man who claims, "When my wife got pregnant, I got pregnant right along with her." During his first month on The Micro Diet he faced a barrage of social eating challenges—three weddings and two anniversary parties. He went to all five events, ate and drank moderately, and still lost seventeen pounds in the month. "I thought to myself, wow, what would happen if I stayed on this diet 'sole source,'" says Stanley. "I did and ended up losing another twenty-five pounds in a month."

Stanley, a thirty-eight-year-old Pittsburgh–based management information systems manager, is now at his goal weight, having shed a total of 125 pounds in eight months. Wife, Peggy, has lost thirty pounds. Says Stanley, "You have to do three things to be successful. Make sure you drink plenty of water. Commit to exercise, and change your eating habits. It's that simple. I have a new body and I intend to keep it that way. I no longer believe that 'diets don't work.' And maintaining one's weight with The Micro Diet is real easy. You just open up the package and eat."

## *BOREDOM*

Probably the dieter's single worst enemy is boredom. You're watching TV and you pop a few peanuts into your mouth. (Ever tried eating just one?) Peanuts are five calories EACH! One packet of potato chips is over 150 calories. Hopefully, your reaction to these rather disturbing facts about the snack industry is glazed shock. In which case, why not pour yourself a glass of one-calorie soda and ponder on the error of *other* people's ways?

If vague visions of a sandwich or potato chips continue to disturb your virtuous thoughts, I urge you to do the following, just once. Get up and go for a walk. Say to yourself, by all means, that you are only doing it to prove me wrong. But when you come back I guarantee you'll feel refreshed, in better spirit, and you may no longer feel hungry. Remember the feeling, and next time you'll go for a walk, not to humor my suggestion, but because you actually found it enjoyable.

## *IF YOU BINGE, DON'T WORRY*

Now here is some advice you never expected. The fact is that we become overweight because of many months (or years) of eating too much, largely the result of some bad habits and poor food choices. You certainly didn't become fat overnight. NOR can you put it all back overnight. As you know, it takes 3,500 calories to produce one pound of fat. So if you gorge yourself on a whole Black Forest gateau, you'll probably gain one pound. Now, because carbohydrate can cause water retention, it will have the effect of temporarily (a day or two) making you weigh as much as three to four pounds heavier, but no further dramatic increase in weight will occur once the body's carbohydrate stores have been filled.

So don't think all is lost. It's just a temporary roadblock in the long-term road to success. If you let one minor lapse put you off the guaranteed route to success, you're being very shortsighted. What you are now doing is laying down a set of lifetime habits. One relapse will make no difference at all.

The same principle applies to eating out. If a friend has invited you out to dine and has put real effort into the meal, or you have a dinner date in a restaurant, you don't have to make a big production about sticking rigidly to a diet. Have something of everything, but be sensible. You can choose the least fattening elements. You can eat small portions of the dessert. That way you emphasize to your subconscious that you are in control. You can have it if you really want it—and this time you decided you really did want it!

In fact, if you're using The Micro Diet "sole source," your calorie intake is so small that you can afford a lapse and probably still be well under your daily calorie expenditure. However, as we've said, eating extra carbohydrates may cause water retention and a weight gain (or slow down in weight loss) that is out of proportion to the actual calories consumed. This is why it is really worth sticking faithfully to the exact program.

## *LISTENING TO YOUR BODY*

Allow your body to tell you what it wants. Now, this doesn't just mean being aware you are full. Sometimes your body seems to cry out for particular foods. If you have a kitchen full of healthy foods, and a fridge full of raw vegetables and fruit juices, and you still crave a Quarter-Pounder, it may well be appropriate to actually go ahead and eat it, as no type of food is forbidden in the loser-friendly program. There is a sound practical reason. Let's suppose you're really craving a big helping of that mud pie in the fridge. Your sensible self says, "Are you mad? There must be seven hundred calories in that!" But the craving persists. "You'd be far better off with a nice raw carrot and a celery snack," says your rational self. But the urge for mud pie persists. So you try to silence it by eating a banana. But the craving is still there.

Well, you've guessed it. In the end, you have the mud pie. So now you've had the raw vegetables, and the banana, and the mud pie. You might as well have had a small piece of the mud pie at the beginning! Denying yourself is only continuing with old-style dieting mentality—and that has failed millions of times.

So is nothing forbidden? Not even the "naughty food"—chocolates for example? No, chocolates if you really want them are OK. When something is forbidden, its attractiveness increases. When you know you can have it, it loses some of its glamour. And it loses some of its glamour when we know why it is such a poor food choice. When you know the full effect some foods have on you, high-sugar foods for example, you can never really feel the same about them. You truly can lose your taste for foods on which you previously binged.

## *THE FIVE-POUND RULE*

Susan Bryan is a firm believer in the five-pound rule. "Never let yourself gain more than five pounds," says Susan, of Langley, British Colombia. "It's much more difficult when you have to face the prospect of losing ten or twelve pounds. I find it's easier to stop yourself at five pounds and to realize that if you don't stop there you may become comfortable gaining larger and larger amounts. Just make the decision that five pounds is your cut-off point, and that's that."

It's a philosophy that Susan has successfully followed for three years since losing fifty-seven pounds in six months, and moving from a size twenty down to a size eleven. Remembers Susan, "I was a package of self-loathing and self-pity wrapped in layers of fat. Today, I have a positive self-image. I can face whatever life throws at me, not with a Pollyanna attitude, but with the realization that I have learned to deal positively with any negative encounters. For the first time I can count on myself. I'm proud of my accomplishment. I can now walk into a room and not wonder if I'm going to be the fattest one there."

Susan feels she used to overeat for a variety of reasons: stress, anger, depression and, in particular, when she was bored. "If I had any free time I would automatically turn to food. Most of the time it was boredom that made me a binge-eater." Today, food plays a secondary role in her life. "I no longer fear the bathroom scale because I can now control what I eat. Visualizing is a very useful technique for me. If I want a piece of pastry, I visualize lard. If I crave something sweet, I visualize five pounds of sugar. Even at a restaurant if I know there's something I shouldn't really be eating, I imagine goblets of fat floating around. It really helps me to see what I'm putting in my body."

Susan, 39, also keeps her weight down through her daily walk. "Maintaining your weight is so much easier when you're active, but it's so important to do something that you enjoy. I like to walk my dog every morning. I walk my son to school as well, and that's great because we have this special time together. I also make a point of parking farther away from places so I can get some additional walking in."

## *BEWARE OF SABOTEURS*

There can be all kinds of people in your life who accidently or otherwise sabotage your efforts to lose weight. Some people may want to show that they care by feeding you. Others may simply not know that you are trying to get rid of your excess fat, or just not appreciate how serious you are. Some may come out with the "Don't you think you're losing too much" attitude because, for whatever reason, they just don't want to see you at your goal weight. It's often said, for instance, that some spouses want their partners to remain overweight so that no one else will find them desirable.

You need to be assertive for your own good. Be polite, but firm. Here are some useful hints: Tell the saboteur that you're trying to lose weight. Stress how important it is to you. Be consistent. Don't say no to a piece of cake one day and then readily accept it the next. Alternatively, you can always take a serving but only eat one or two bites, or take it, saying you'll save it for later (and then give or throw it away). Keep in mind the fact that if you do allow someone to force you into eating something you don't want because you're afraid of hurting their feelings, you'll probably end up resenting that person or blaming yourself.

Practice your responses for those occasions when people try to force you to eat, e.g., "I can't eat another bite. I'm trying to watch my weight. MY DOCTOR INSISTS I LOSE WEIGHT." If all else fails, avoid the saboteur.

## *MAKE A FRESH START— FORGET THE OLD-STYLE DIET MENTALITY*

The reason many diets fail is that they ask you to make too many changes too fast. The all or nothing approach nearly always ends up as nothing. The whole theme of the loser-friendly program is to give you a wide variety of choices involving a series of individually minor changes that add up to success. None of the individual changes involves much effort, but together they accumulate to a major and decisive change.

The first thing that's wrong with old-style diets is that they emphasize "Don't!" If you are told not to do something—what is the very thing that you start thinking about? The typical old-style dieter will deny himself. Do without breakfast and skip lunch. So far, he feels virtuous. But then once home, he is feeling desperately hungry. So food begins to loom large in his mind. In an entirely mistaken impression that he is exercising will-power, he tries to resist eating. So by the time he does start to eat, you can bet he'll eat the wrong foods, and too fast. In the end he'll eat far more than he ever would have done with a more relaxed approach. The likely result is that he'll then feel over-fed, guilty, and quite possibly abandon the whole thing as not worthwhile. That vicious circle all started because he started with the old-style diet mentality—concentrating on what NOT to do, using misguided will-power instead of common sense.

In contrast, I believe the ONLY way to succeed is to acknowledge that food is there to be enjoyed and "you can have it if you really want it." But there is the rub. Do you really want it? Now, clearly, you must be willing to answer the question realistically. If you ask the question while you're holding a second helping of chocolate cake in your hand the answer is likely to be "yes!" You need to be able to answer the question under more objective circumstances. For example:

1. You are at the table. Do you really want an extra helping? Wait five minutes. Be aware of how your body feels. Then

answer. If you still want more, go ahead and enjoy it. You decided consciously to eat it rather than automatically starting on the second helping—and you should relish it.

2. You walk into the kitchen and see some leftover cake. Don't just wolf it down. You can have it if you really want it, but do you really want it? Walk out again and do something for the next ten minutes. Now decide.
3. You are at a restaurant. The waiter asks if you want dessert. Remember, you can have it if you really want it. Say you'll let him know in a minute or two. Get up from the table and go to the rest room. Now you are removed from the environment when the automatic unthinking reaction is to continue with a dessert. Given the short break you will now probably become aware that you actually feel pretty full. There is a good chance when you return to the table you can genuinely say, "No, on reflection I really don't want dessert."
4. You are relaxing in the evening and you feel like eating chocolate. A few pieces is hardly a disaster, so you can have it if you really want. Now, if you've been taking note of the advice in this book, there will be none in the house. (Because if it isn't immediately available you can't immediately eat it.) So now the question is, "Do I really want it, and do I want it enough to go to the store for it?" That's an instructive question.
5. You are at home over the weekend and the kids are screaming for hamburger and fries. It sounds like a good idea to you, too. Fair enough. You know enough to grill the Quarter-Pounder rather than fry it, and to use the large fries because they absorb less fat, but do you really want it? You busy yourself, wait five minutes, and decide that you do want it.

Now's the time to learn to be a "calorie trader." A calorie trader is someone who is quite happy to trade a little exercise for some favorite food. So you estimate that the favorite treat is around 600 calories. Walking briskly burns up about four calories a minute. So the question is, do you want it enough to trade it for a 150-minute walk?

Now, this question not only helps highlight the point of whether you really want the meal, it is an excellent way of making calories a meaningful measurement. It's quite fun, and definitely educational, to express food not only in calories but in "exercise equivalents." Why not play the game yourself, converting your favorite foods into minutes of walking? (One minute walking =four to five calories burnt.)

Here are a few examples:

| | Calories Involved | Minutes of Walking to Burn Up Calories |
|---|---|---|
| 2 slices of toast with butter and marmalade or jam | 365 | 73–91 minutes |
| 1 corned beef sandwich | 370 | 74–93 minutes |
| 1 pkg. peanuts (2 ounces) | 325 | 65–81 minutes |
| 1 pkg. potato chips (2 ounces) | 305 | 61–76 minutes |
| 1 granola bar (2 ounces) | 110 | 22–28 minutes |
| 2 pancakes | 275 | 55–69 minutes |
| 1 chocolate Mr. Goodbar | 300 | 60–75 minutes |
| Ice cream (3 ounces) | 140 | 28–35 minutes |
| 1 cup hot chocolate | 240 | 48–60 minutes |
| 1 bottle beer (12 ounces) | 150 | 30–37 minutes |
| 1 ounce cheddar cheese and Wheat Thins | 260 | 52–68 minutes |
| 1 large chocolate chip cookie | 200 | 40–50 minutes |

Let me make a suggestion. Next time you do decide "I really do want that extra," go ahead, but first walk it off. You'll enjoy the walk, you'll feel a lot more relaxed, and you'll enjoy that "extra" all the more.

## *A RECAP*

Let's take a break and review what we have learned:

1. Many overweight people really do gain weight easily. They eat more than their body can currently metabolize, but they don't necessarily overeat compared with other people.
2. Most people eat for psychological reasons as well as to satisfy their physical needs. Unfortunately, the person who puts on weight easily finds that his or her body just can't cope with those extra calories, so he can't afford to feed his mind as well as his body.

3. Calories certainly count. It's wise to know the foods that have a well-above-average fattening effect. That knowledge will genuinely influence our attitude toward them. We can cook and eat to de-emphasize them.
4. Old-style dieting and denial is counter-productive. You know and I know that it is not that simple. What's needed is a positive program that's realistic, enjoyable, and which works.

The loser-friendly program works. It partly involves common sense and partly involves putting into practice a number of minor changes. None of them is individually difficult, but they can add up to a dramatic effect on your life.

# 15

# TRUE OR FALSE?

IT REALLY IS AMAZING how popular mythology can take hold. In the diet and nutrition arena, in particular, so many misunderstandings seem to abound. Here's a fun test, which is extremely instructive at the same time.

**T/F Carbohydrates have fewer calories per gram than fat.**
**A:** True. One gram of fat contains nine calories. One gram of carbohydrate or protein has only four.

**T/F Fresh vegetables provide the best nutrition.**
**A:** False. Vegetables often lose their nutrients between the farm and your grocer through being shipped long distance, exposure to sun, and sitting around in produce bins. Quick-frozen vegetables are often more nutritious.

**T/F "Light" foods always contain fewer calories.**
**A:** False. The whole question of food labelling is currently under review, but some manufacturers have used the term "light" to mean that the product tastes light, not that it is lower in calories, fat, or sodium! Read the label carefully.

**T/F Margarine is less caloric than butter.**
**A:** False. Both have exactly 100 calories per tablespoon.

**T/F Grapefruit is great to eat on a diet because it will "burn off" the fat.**
**A:** False. Grapefruit is not a magic fat burner. To successfully lose weight you must reduce your caloric intake.

**T/F French fries have less sodium than a vanilla milk shake.**

A: True. A typical "fast food" vanilla shake has 200 mg of sodium and an average order of French fries contains only 109 mg of sodium.

**T/F You can depend on "health foods" to provide good nutrition.**

A: False. Many health foods such as banana chips and granola bars are loaded with sugar and fat.

**T/F Fighting fat should be more important to women than to men.**

A: False. Only half as many men as women in the United States are dieting, yet it is the apple-shape weight that accumulates more frequently in the upper torso and abdomen in men, which is more dangerous from a health standpoint.

**T/F A wine cooler is a good alcoholic beverage to drink while dieting, as it is low in calories.**

A: False. At 200 calories per twelve-ounce serving, wine coolers are more fattening than beer, which has only 155 calories for the same size serving.

**T/F Eating salad is a surefire way to lose weight.**

A: False. A chef's salad can contain up to 1,000 calories. Skip the meat and rich dressings. Stick to vegetables and reduced-calorie dressings.

**T/F Two percent milk is not really low fat.**

A: True. The Center for Science in the Public Interest says that 2% milk should not be considered low fat, for it contains almost as much fat as whole milk (3.3% butterfat).

**T/F Brown rice is better for you than white rice.**

A: False. Enriched white rice has about the same nutritional value as brown rice. Brown rice does, however, have more fiber.

**T/F Fruit drinks and fruit juices are the same product.**

A: False. Unless a product contains 100% real fruit juice, it must be labeled as a drink. A "fruit drink" may have just 10–34% juice.

**T/F Brown sugar and honey are better for you than white sugar.**
**A:** False. They all contain similar, insignificant amounts of micro-nutrients.

**T/F Some sugar-coated cereals are better for you than granola.**
**A:** True. Granola can be considerably higher in calories, fat, and sugar than most cereals.

**T/F "All natural" foods do not contain additives.**
**A:** False. Many additives are derived from natural sources.

**T/F Preservative-free foods may not be as healthy for you as those with preservatives.**
**A:** True. Preservatives help protect your food from rancidity, mold growth, insect infestation, and loss of important vitamins. Also, some preservatives even have direct health benefits.

**T/F Vegetable oils which state "no cholesterol" on their labels are better for you than those which don't.**
**A:** False. Neither contain cholesterol since it is only found in animal products.

**T/F Foods which are "unsalted" or have "no salt added" do not contain salt.**
**A:** False. These statements indicate that no salt was added in making a product which normally contains salt. This product may contain sodium from additives as well as other sources. Don't be fooled.

**T/F Children do not need to worry about high cholesterol.**
**A:** False. Two-thirds of the children in the United States have a cholesterol level above 150.

**T/F Some vegetables have twice as much vitamin C as an orange and only half the number of calories.**
**A:** True. Many fresh vegetables such as green peppers, broccoli, cauliflower, and Brussels sprouts have more vitamin C with a lot less calories and sugar than an orange.

**T/F A gram of protein and a gram of carbohydrate have the same number of calories.**
**A:** True. They both have four calories per gram, but you

are likely to have your appetite satisfied with fewer calories from carbohydrates.

T/F **A high-protein diet is necessary for good muscle tone.**
**A:** False. Muscles will be no stronger or better on a high-protein diet than on one which supplies the Recommended Dietary Allowance (RDA).

T/F **I should completely eliminate salt from my diet.**
**A:** False. Sodium is important for the proper functioning of your body, for salt is the base mineral in the blood.

T/F **Hormone problems, particularly thyroid deficiencies, are often responsible for many cases of obesity.**
**A:** False. Although this statement was once believed by health professionals, recent evidence suggests that only a very small percentage of weight problems are influenced by hormone imbalances.

# 16

# YOUR QUESTIONS ANSWERED

IT'S YOUR BODY, and your life. And anyone embarking on a weight-loss program should thoroughly examine the program from a very personal perspective. I've compiled for you every question about the diet that I've been asked over the last decade.

**Is it necessary to take additional vitamins and minerals while on this plan?**

No! As long as you have at least three Micro meals a day you are receiving at least 100% of the Recommended Dietary Allowances. If you are enjoying just two Micro meals and a well-balanced regular meal it is likely that you will be receiving all the nutrition that you need. However, the choice is yours. If you do wish to supplement your diet, for some specific reason, ask your doctor.

**Will everyone lose weight on this diet? I've tried everything and nothing seems to work.**

Yes! Everyone should lose weight if they faithfully follow the instructions. The only difference is how much and how fast. No one, over a period of time, can maintain their weight on the sole souce of nutrition program which provides 800 calories a day. There has to be a continued FAT loss, even if the scales don't indicate weight loss. In general, nature makes men burn more calories than women, therefore men lose faster.

### Why are pregnant women advised not to go on the diet?

Generally speaking, they should not be on any diet—after all they're eating for two. Mothers-to-be should plan their diet carefully and always seek their physician's advice. The metabolic changes which occur by reducing one's caloric intake to as little as 800 calories a day may have an undesirable impact on the fetus. Pregnant women are also usually prescribed extra vitamins and it would not be wise to take unnecessary supplements.

### Will this diet program benefit my arthritis?

The plan will not cure any type of arthritis, but arthritic symptoms of the weight-bearing joints will probably be alleviated *by the loss of excess weight.* Patients frequently report that they are able to decrease the amount of anti-inflammatory drugs. Some claim total freedom from any symptoms.

### I have diabetes. Is the diet OK for me?

The medical experts familiar with low-calorie diets feel that this is an excellent method for the treatment of Type II diabetes—obese maturity onset diabetes. This is the most prevalent form of diabetes, comprising more than 90% of all cases in the United States. There are many case histories in which all clinical evidence of diabetes disappears as the patient approaches his or her ideal weight. Patients must be under the direct supervision of a physician as medication will almost certainly need to be reduced or eliminated.

People who have Type I diabetes, which usually begins in childhood or adolescence and always necessitates insulin treatment, are rarely overweight. For those individuals who are overweight, constantly adjusting insulin dosages to match reduced caloric intake is extremely complex, should seldom be tried and, if tried, should only be with strict and careful physician supervision.

### Why do you recommend drinking so much liquid every day?

Water is good for you. Our bodies consist of over 60% water, so we need to constantly replace our body fluids. Sufficient liquid intake is also required to keep our kidneys functioning properly and to help prevent constipation.

**Could I take the liquid in the form of beer or other kinds of alcohol?**

Only if you want to get drunk really fast. Seriously, alcohol is a major impediment to any diet plan. It contains seven calories per gram compared with four calories per gram of protein or carbohydrate. In fact, it almost holds as many calories as fat, which "costs" nine calories per gram.

But there may be even more to it than the number of calories per gram. A 1992 study, published in the *New England Journal of Medicine*, reported that when you drink alcohol, your body burns fat much more slowly than usual. Swiss researchers at the University of Zurich found that people who consumed the equivalent of six shots of whiskey or six beers a day reduced their body's burning of fat by one-third. Just why this happens is unclear.

**What about coffee?**

Be careful. It's amazing the number of calories you can accumulate if you add milk and sugar. Typically, the addition of milk and two teaspoons of sugar would provide an extra fifty-nine calories.

**What about soda drinks?**

Avoid them like the plague! They're full of calories and have little or no nutritional content. A can of Coke, for instance, has 130 calories.

**Are diet sodas permissible then?**

Yes, you're on safer ground here, as most only contain one calorie per serving.

**Why is there so much sodium in the Micro meals?**

The diet is formulated to provide all of the necessary nutrients for someone on a weight-loss program. The amount of sodium per meal varies from 80 mg in the popcorn bar to 850 mg in the chicken soup. On average, a dieter enjoying three Micro meals a day would consume no more than 1,500 mg of sodium, which is generally considered quite low. The U.S. *Surgeon General's Report on Nutrition and Health* states that, for adults, a safe and adequate daily intake of sodium is between 1,100 mg and 3,300 mg. The American Heart Association recommends a maximum of 3,000 mg per day. Sodium is an essential element, and a sodium/potassium balance is particularly important. Unfortunately, the general discussion about the need to limit sodium intake sometimes creates the impression it is not needed. Note: one teaspoon of salt contains 2,000 mg of sodium. A McDonald's Big Mac contains 1,510 mg of sodium.

**Won't I become constipated if I only consume 800 calories a day?**

It depends on what you mean by constipation. If much less bulk is being consumed, you should not expect to be as regular as you were before you started the diet. This is perfectly normal and no cause for concern. However, it is quite permissible to add fiber to your daily intake, always bearing in mind the calories you will also be adding. You may prefer to avoid extra calories by adding natural bran or commercial preparations such as sugarless Metamucil. A greater potential for constipation exists if sufficient fluid is not consumed, so it is important to follow our recommended intake of fluids a day. The vast majority of dieters tend to choose at least two higher calorie Micro meals a day that contain fiber (such as the bars) and, therefore, they do not report any problems with constipation.

**Soon after starting the diet I developed a bad cold. Why was this?**

You caught a cold virus. It's as simple as that. You've had colds in the past and you will certainly catch a cold in the future. It was just an unfortunate coincidence.

**I'm worried that by losing a lot of weight quickly, I will look gaunt and haggard. Are you sure this won't happen?**

On the contrary, people who lose weight with The Micro Diet often tell us that they feel healthy and look healthy. The drawn look usually occurs when people have been starving themselves or have lost weight through illness. With this program you're not depriving yourself of anything—except calories.

**If I find it difficult to use The Micro Diet as my sole source of nutrition can I take an appetite suppressant?**

It is strongly recommended that you don't. Appetite suppressants can cause unpleasant side effects such as headaches, anxiety, and even nausea. Even worse, amphetamines, for instance, are highly addictive and can have an adverse effect on the heart and central nervous system. The truth of the matter is that appetite suppressants are just not necessary. If you experience any mild hunger pangs they will disappear after the first few days.

**What happens if I can't resist temptation and I "cheat" while I'm on the diet?**

This is the benevolent diet. Since your basic calorie intake is so low, having a snack or adding a meal will, at worst, halt your weight-loss pattern for a day or so. Once you are back on one of the Loser-Friendly plans you'll start shedding fat again. Whatever happens, continue with three or four Micro meals every day. Chances are that as long as you do that you'll succeed; you'll be so satisfied that you won't feel the need for so many other foods.

**What is the role of exercise in your diet plan?**

Moderate exercise is certainly important to help your muscle tone and cardiovascular function. However, do not start a rigorous exercise program at the same time you start the diet. This will be too much of a strain for your body. Take a look at the "Stefanie Powers' Broadway Workout." It was designed for the overweight person and beginner. Exercise is fully discussed in Chapter Twelve.

**Is it all right to take tranquillizers when I'm dieting?**

There are no known contra-indications, but if you are taking any kind of medication whatsoever you are strongly advised to discuss it when you consult your doctor.

**Is there any way to get rid of fat faster from specific areas?**

As long as you're consuming just 800 calories a day on The Micro Diet you will keep losing fat. There is no way of controlling target areas other than through surgical procedures. Various gimmicks and devices have been promoted but have no clinical substantiation for their claims.

**I've been told that the only way I can really lose 100 extra pounds is through surgery. What do you think?**

Try The Micro Diet first. An operation such as gastroplasty, or stomach stapling, should be a last-resort treatment.

**I want to stay on the program as my "sole source" of nutrition for longer than the recommended three weeks. Can I?**

Hospital patients have remained on this kind of low-calorie, nutritionally complete diet for months at a time. However, we insist that three consecutive weeks of "sole source" be observed, alternated with an "add-a-meal" week to help in the re-education of food habits, and because each individual is different. Also, it is worth bearing in mind that although all of the nutrients that are known to science are included in Micro meals, there is always the remote possibility that there is some element present in other foods which is not obtainable through these nutritionally enhanced meals or a multi-vitamin pill.

**Doesn't this kind of diet cause diarrhea?**

A very small number of people might experience this reaction as a result of the mineral content of the meals. Taking in extra liquids will reduce the problem. If diarrhea persists for more than two or three days, the diet should be temporarily discontinued and your doctor consulted. It may be that you have a lactose intolerance—milk is the primary source of protein in some of the meals.

**I suffer from high blood pressure. Is the diet OK for me?**

A patient's blood pressure is usually lowered once they are successfully losing weight and this is aided by the low sodium content and diuretic effect. Therefore, it is likely that anyone taking antihypertensive medication will need the dosage decreased. That's why it's important that no one with hypertension start the diet without a physician's advice and frequent blood pressure checks. The patient should never "prescribe" for himself or herself.

**Is the low-calorie diet suitable for the elderly?**

Yes, for the obese elderly, particularly those with a medical problem such as adult-onset diabetes, arthritis, or high blood pressure, the diet plan, used under medical supervision, could be quite beneficial.

**Can my overweight 12-year-old son lose weight with this plan?**

Low-calorie diets, per se, are not recommended for growing

children, but substituting the Micro drinks for regular milk shakes, ice cream, etc., or a Micro bar instead of a candy bar, makes a good alternative for your offspring.

**Can a mother use the diet while breast-feeding?**

Not as the sole source of nutrition, but certainly as a nutritional supplement. Micro meals contain all of the vitamins and minerals necessary to promote good health in both mother and child. A new mother will obviously be medically monitored.

**How soon can a new mother, who is not breast-feeding, start seriously dieting?**

This is a decision for her doctor, although normally a waiting period of two weeks would be sufficient.

**What do I do if I've had my three or four Micro meals and still find that I'm hungry?**

This is really only likely to happen during the first few days on the diet plan. Later, you may not have any cravings at all. To counteract hunger pangs, help yourself to an extra Micro meal. You will be getting much better value from those calories than from any other snack. You really do have to ask yourself where you're feeling hungry—your stomach or your head?

**Isn't there a danger that I could consume too many vitamins and minerals by having extra Micro meals?**

Three Micro meals provide entirely sufficient nutrition for most people's needs. An extra meal is permissible as most vitamins are water soluble and are simply passed through the body if not needed.

**Could I become anemic on this diet plan?**

There is no evidence whatsoever that anemia could be a side effect. A woman who suffers heavy and prolonged menstrual periods should bear in mind that a potential for anemia exists, even when she is not on a weight-loss plan.

**Can I give blood while on the rapid weight-loss program?**

Ask the blood bank what their rules are. It's probably not a good idea to give blood while on any kind of weight-loss plan because it would reduce your blood volume and could aggravate postural hypotension (you would feel dizzy when standing up quickly).

**I usually become more depressed when I'm dieting. What do you suggest?**

Most studies have shown that overweight people are no more or less depressed than the rest of the population. Our experience is that during the active dieting phase of the program, the dieter's mood is a reflection of their success. Someone losing their weight is likely to be ecstatic; a dieter who, for some reason is not succeeding, will become frustrated and possibly depressed. Someone who is under health care for severe depression may well find that their doctor feels that the stress of a diet plan is too much for them, or will want to constantly monitor the situation. Once again, ask your doctor.

**It occurs to me that the low-calorie regimen might make me anorexic. Could this happen?**

Absolutely not. Anorexia nervosa is a largely misunderstood condition. It is a phobia—a severe psychiatric problem. Drastically reducing one's calorie intake as part of a diet plan will not, in itself, lead to anorexia nervosa. We do, however, feel strongly that dieters should aim to be healthy and attractively slim, but not thin. Teenage girls should not be on a low-calorie weight-loss program. A few pounds overweight represents much less of a health hazard than obsessive dieting.

**I have a tendency toward gout. What do you advise?**

People with gout usually have a higher level of uric acid in their blood. The problem with many diets is that they increase the uric acid level, which can precipitate gouty attacks. This would almost certainly occur during the first few days on the diet and medication might be required. In those people who remain on the diet, the uric acid level eventually comes back down to its pre-existing state. People with established gout should go on a low-calorie diet only with their doctor's specific recommendation and monitoring. People with high uric acid levels should also be under medical supervision as they may need medication.

**I know that potassium is important for my heart. Is there really enough in The Micro Diet?**

For the normal person who is not taking diuretics (water pills) or other medication, there is sufficient potassium. Clinical studies have not indicated any evidence of potassium depletion with dieters on nutritionally complete, low-calorie diets containing similar amounts of potassium to The Micro Diet. It is imperative that people taking medication, particularly for high blood pressure, consult their doctor so that he or she can monitor potassium levels, and supplement if necessary.

**I've had a heart attack and I know I need to lose a lot of weight, but isn't your diet too stressful for me?**

Many heart patients have had positive experiences with low-calorie diets. But I must emphasize that this is a matter for the judgment of the individual physician, and constant monitoring would be necessary. No one with a serious medical condition should embark on any diet program without the total approval of his or her doctor. In particular, it's important to mention stroke victims and patients with kidney and liver ailments.

**What is ketosis and am I likely to get it?**

Ketone bodies are derived from the breakdown of fat and indicate that the body is consuming its fat stores. More severe ketosis is often caused by high-protein, low-carbohydrate, badly balanced diets. The Micro Diet is formulated to give a very specific balance of carbohydrate as well as protein. There is a moderate rise in ketone levels in people using a low-calorie diet. Ketone bodies may suppress appetite which is one reason why the dieter doesn't feel hungry, but does feel well.

**I find that I have bad breath. Why?**

A small number of dieters report experiencing halitosis or bad breath. In some cases this may be due to the production of ketones and in others it is caused by a reduction in saliva or the reflux of gas from the stomach. Drinking plenty of fluids speeds up stomach emptying and also helps to wash the mouth.

**I am taking special medication. Is that a problem?**

Repeat: Ask your doctor.

**I suffer from acute gall bladder attacks. Is it safe to use this diet?**

There is no evidence to indicate that this specific program would cause gall bladder problems. However, by being overweight in the first instance, your risk for gall stone formation is three to four times greater than for non-obese individuals. In addition, it is important to note that there is a fair amount of cholesterol stored in body fat. When one goes on a low-calorie diet this is mobilized with increased cholesterol secretion in the bile. This, in turn, may slightly increase the risks for forming gall stones. Most of the evidence indicating this potential comes from studies of diets containing no more than 500 calories a day. The Micro Diet, of course, is a minimum of 800 calories a day. Anyone who has a documented history of gall bladder attacks should not embark on any low-calorie diet. Micro meals can, however, be used as a part of a more modest reduced calorie intake.

**Am I too heavy to exercise?**

It doesn't matter how overweight you are, you can always start slowly, spending just a few minutes a day on a non-strenuous routine. Walking is an excellent activity. Read Chapter Twelve and definitely look at the "Stefanie Powers' Broadway Workout" tape. You'll find people of all shapes and sizes having a great time as they work out.

**I find that I don't need as much sleep when I'm on the "sole source" plan. Is this usual?**

Quite often dieters report that they are up and running much earlier in the mornings. Overeating has a definite sedative effect. So dieting itself, balanced nutrition, and increased vitality may combine to cut the hours of sleep you require. Spend your extra time wisely!

**Does The Micro Diet contain any preservatives?**

There are no preservatives, drugs, or diuretics in any of our meals. They are natural foods supplemented with vitamins, minerals, trace elements, and electrolytes.

**Will dieting hurt my sex life?**

On the contrary. Many people enthusiastically comment on a new "frisky" attitude. It's not surprising really, when you realize the increased physical vigor and mental self-enhancement which accompanies weight loss.

**This diet sounds too good to be true. There must be some negative side effects.**

As with any weight-loss program your body is undergoing a dramatic change in routine and may react in many different ways. A very small minority of people may experience some problems which are usually mild and last just a day or two. The long-term benefits make them more than worthwhile. With an 800-calorie-a-day plan, however, we have found far fewer reports of minor side effects such as headaches, dizziness, and nausea than encountered with lower calorie intakes. Headaches may occur because of withdrawal from caffeine to which your body has become addicted, or through not taking enough fluid. The solution is to drink plenty of water. Dizziness, especially when standing up quickly, can result from the diuretic effect that accompanies any low-calorie diet. Again the remedy is to drink plenty of fluids (and don't stand up quickly). Additional salt intake can be extremely useful—try bouillon. Some people may initially react to the high concentration of nutrients in the Micro meals by feeling nauseous. This is a very temporary condition. It can also be alleviated by drinking extra water. If this is not effective, eat normally, adding the meals as a supplement and then gradually discontinue the other foods.

**I have a sweet tooth. Can I add artificial sweetener to the drinks?**

It's entirely up to you. Many people find, however, that they seem to have much less desire for sweet things when consuming The Micro Diet.

**I've been told that it's not a good idea to boil the soups. Why is that?**

If you mix the soup powder with water and then bring to the boil, you will be cooking away some of the vital nutrients, especially vitamins. If you use a blender, always add the powder to hot water; if you mix it by hand, add the product to a little cold water and mix to make a smooth paste, then add the rest of the water. Eat it within the next ten minutes or so.

**Should I continue with the diet if I catch the flu?**

It's not advisable to be losing weight while you're sick. Wait until you've recovered.

**I am going through the "change of life." Is the diet suitable for me?**

Yes. There's no reason why menopause should hold you back from getting your body in tip-top shape. The diet plan should be a positive step at this stage of your life, making you look and feel better. We have encountered women who have found they experience fewer hot flashes while on the diet.

**Does it matter how many fat cells I have? Do they increase when I get fatter?**

An adult has anywhere from twenty to sixty billion fat cells with an average of around forty billion. Some obese individuals have two to three times the normal number. The increase in the number of fat cells generally occurs during childhood and adolescence. There is not much increase after the age of 18 to 20. In becoming overweight there is a significant enlargement in fat cell size—they can even, reportedly, swell to as much as three times their normal size. By losing weight the size of the fat cells will reduce toward a normal size—but there is no good evidence to suggest that you'll lose any of the fat cells themselves. You're stuck with them.

**I need to gain weight, so I guess your program is not for me.**

Wrong. By enjoying Micro meals as a supplement to other food you'll be adding extra protein, vitamins, and minerals.

**Is it normal to feel so thirsty when I'm dieting?**

Sometimes when people are thirsty, it's simply their body's way of telling them that it needs more fluids. Simply drink more water. It's good for you. In fact, you shouldn't really wait until your body is crying out for water. Liquid is an essential part of the diet plan.

**Is there enough fiber in The Micro Diet?**

Three or four Micro meals provide up to thirty-two grams of fiber a day. If a greater amount of fiber is desired, the dieter should take natural bran, a commercial preparation, or eat fruit and vegetables (watch the calories, though). However, you should also bear in mind that all of the clinical research has indicated no serious ill effects from short-term usage of a low-calorie diet devoid of fiber. There is a full section on fiber in Chapter Two.

**Why is The Micro Diet not sold in drug stores?**

Because the advice, support, and encouragement of the Independent Micro Diet Advisor is an integral part of the program.

**When I reach my ideal weight I intend to celebrate by going out for a big feast. Is this OK?**

Celebrate with caution. It is not a wise move to suddenly overload your system after it has become used to a low-calorie regimen. Do not eat a large meal after a period on the 800-calorie-a-day plan. This will be too stressful for your digestive system.

**So, does every member of the medical profession endorse a low-calorie diet?**

As more and more clinical studies on low-calorie diets find their way into the medical literature, greater numbers of scientists are becoming convinced that this method of weight loss really is the answer. Those doctors who question the validity of low-calorie diets usually make the following points:

1. The diet should be medically supervised. (I feel that anyone commencing any weight-loss program should first consult with his or her doctor.)
2. It's important to teach people better eating habits. (That's what half of this book is about, and that's why we have produced the *Choices* lifestyle modification program.)
3. There's a danger of the dieter losing muscle tissue and protein from vital organs. (The most recent evidence shows that the amount of protein lost on a nutritionally complete, low-calorie diet is only to be expected as protein, as well as fat, constitutes the weight that had been gained.)

**Why do some people feel cold when they are dieting?**

When people reduce their food intake the body reduces its energy/heat output so, unless they wear more clothes (or move to Florida), they will tend to feel cold.

**Are menstrual irregularities a side effect of the diet?**

Occasionally, some women do notice menstrual irregularities and this is due to the change in body weight. When the weight stabilizes, the cycle returns to normal. Some overweight women fail to menstruate, but when they lose weight the periods return.

**I sometimes experience leg cramps when I am on the diet. Why is this?**

It is possible that this may arise from losing too much salt from the body. The Micro Diet is relatively low in salt and that may be a contributory factor. If cramping occurs, a little extra salt should be added to the diet.

**Why do you lose water when you diet?**

When you diet you obviously reduce your intake of calories. This will mean that initially the body is using up part of its store of glycogen. Since each gram of glycogen in the body binds with four grams of water, when the glycogen is burnt up as energy, it releases four grams of water (and some sodium as well). Conversely, when people who have used up their glycogen stores "binge" on carbohydrate they will notice a rapid weight gain of up to three to four pounds because the glycogen stores are once again filled...with both glycogen and water.

**Why do ex-smokers gain weight?**

It's not necessarily because they turn to food for comfort and eat more—although that may certainly be a contributory factor! The latest studies show that smoking increases metabolic rate, helping to burn up more calories—as much as a hundred calories per day, which is equivalent to a one-mile walk. When they quit smoking the average person, even if they eat the same as before, will gain at least one pound a month until they put on at least five to ten additional pounds in weight.

Giving up the cigarettes is a major accomplishment for anyone, as smoking is undoubtedly a much bigger health hazard than obesity. Dr. Kenneth A. Perkins, who conducted a major smoking study, says nonsmokers "would have to gain more than fifty pounds to be at the same risk of cancer and heart disease as smokers." Unfortunately, that does happen. The message is clear: Give up smoking and make a specific adjustment in your eating habits at the same time.

### Is there much cholesterol in The Micro Diet?

There is very little cholesterol, if any, in The Micro Diet. The peanut, crunchy peanut, popcorn, and yogurt-orange bars, the hearty pea soup, and the chili contain no cholesterol at all. Very little cholesterol is found in the shakes and soups—only ten milligrams per serving in the vanilla, chocolate, and strawberry drinks, and the creamy chicken soup. Five milligrams of cholesterol are included in each serving of muesli cereal and the tetrazzini meal. The creamy tomato soup has four milligrams. By comparison, just one egg yolk contains 252 milligrams of cholesterol, one tablespoon of butter has thirty-five milligrams, one cup of whole milk contains thirty-four milligrams, three ounces of scallops have forty-five milligrams, and three ounces of white turkey (no skin) contain sixty-five milligrams.

### Is The Micro Diet FDA approved?

There is considerable public confusion over the role of the FDA. The Micro Diet is a food product and, as such, is not inspected by the FDA before manufacture. However, the FDA has power to take action should the product be mislabelled or its use misrepresented in any way. Micro Diet products have been manufactured in accordance with the rules of all regulatory agencies. The Micro Diet has been sold in the United States since June 1987 with no complaint from the FDA.

### What is the shelf life of Micro Diet products and are there any special storage recommendations?

The Micro drinks, soups, and international cuisine meals have a shelf life of at least eighteen months. The bars and muesli have a shelf life of at least nine months. It is recommended that Micro Diet products be stored in a cool, dry, hygienic area, at least four inches off the floor. Bars, in particular, should be kept at seventy degrees or cooler.

### Is there any reason why a dieter should not eat three Micro bars a day?

The protein content of most of the Micro bars is fifteen grams per serving and therefore, if one's sole source of calories is three Micro bars a day then this would amount to forty-five grams of protein. Although providing the RDA of protein for women (forty-four grams), it does not meet the RDA for men (fifty-six grams). Over a one-week period, for instance, this decrease in protein intake is not likely to have a harmful effect, but prolonged intake at this level is not recommended. We suggest that the Micro bars be intermixed with the other products to keep the protein intake up, as well as to provide a more varied and flavorful diet program.

### I have heard that losing weight on a low-calorie diet will "mess up" my metabolism. Is that right?

No. However, some perfectly normal changes do occur as your body adapts to the lower calorie intake. After a few days there is a 10% to 20% reduction in the basal metabolic rate (the number of calories burned just sitting around). This lowering of the metabolic rate is a sensible, normal response. In a way, it's the body's "defense mechanism" at work. After all, in a situation of food shortage or famine, the body needs to be able to reduce its caloric needs in order to enhance survival.

In America today, of course, caloric deprivation in healthy people is usually a conscious decision involving dieting, and the body's built-in response works against the dieter, slowing down the rate of weight loss. Don't be discouraged. For most dieters the small reduction in the rate of weight loss will make little difference in the time it takes to reach the ultimate goal weight.

The precise cause of this lower metabolic rate is not completely understood, but is at least partly due to a decrease in thyroid hormone levels. The hormones produced by the thyroid gland are important in controlling your metabolic rate. When an individual who has been on a low-calorie diet resumes eating normally, the adaptive responses reverse, and the metabolic rate returns to normal over a period of several days.

Consuming a normal amount of calories, however, while the body is still running at a somewhat reduced metabolic rate, may cause weight gain. For this reason, it is wise to gradually resume normal caloric intake after a period of dieting to keep pace with the body's gradual readjustment to normal metabolic rate. It is important to understand that none of the adaptive changes in metabolic rate are permanent and all are readily and completely reversed when normal calorie intake is resumed.

**Is it true that when you lose weight rapidly on a low-calorie diet you lose vital lean body tissue?**

Lean body tissue is defined as any body component other than fat, and therefore consists of protein, fluid, carbohydrate stores, and other minor components. When individuals go on complete starvation diets or consume very low-calorie diets without protein, or even with low-quality protein, body tissue is broken down. However, many recent studies have shown that when adequate amounts of high-quality protein are ingested daily (values range from forty to seventy grams per day), low-calorie diets can be safely consumed without excessive loss of protein body mass.

Despite these findings, skeptics have stated that it is always possible that a small amount of protein is lost from some critical tissue or body compartment which may be important to normal functioning. Despite numerous studies, no definite evidence for this idea has surfaced.

**When I read the Micro Diet packaging it looks as if the products are full of chemicals. What's the story?**

Those chemical sounding words are actually just the proper scientific declaration for the nature-identical nutrients, e.g., pyridoxine hydrochloride is vitamin B6.

**Can someone taking steroids use The Micro Diet?**

There are two classes of steroids. There is the kind that immediately springs into many people's minds and that's anabolic steroids, the type of illegal steroid that football players and other athletes get caught cheating on. They are illegal and obviously out of bounds. The other kind of steroid is cortisone or prednisone, an anti-inflammatory drug given to patients for a variety of medical conditions. When people are taking this kind of steroid they should not be on a low-calorie diet, because one of the effects of the steroid is to break down body protein. In combination with a low-calorie diet this might lead to an excessive loss of lean body tissue.

**Is it harder for women taking an estrogen replacement to lose weight?**

Women who are deficient in estrogen (i.e., women who have

had ovaries removed or are post-menopausal) are prone to gain weight. However, taking an estrogen replacement brings their hormones back to normal and, therefore, they should not have any increased difficulty in losing weight.

# 17

# WHAT YOU'VE LEARNED

CONGRATULATIONS. You've made it to the last chapter of the book. You're on the homeward stretch. You've learned a lot, enough to help you make some important changes in your life, so that you can lose weight and keep it off. Now that you've discovered what the loser-friendly Micro Diet is all about, I've used Loser-Friendly as an acronym to help you remember the key points of this program.

**L**ong-lasting
**O**ptional
**S**afe
**E**asy
**R**apid

**F**illing
**R**ealistic
**I**ntegrity
**E**ffective
**N**utritious
**D**elicious
**L**ife-changing
**Y**ou're never alone

## *LONG-LASTING*

The loser-friendly Micro Diet works. All of the evidence indicates that following this program represents your best chance—

not only to lose the excess weight, but also for permanent results. You've met many of our long-term winners at losing in the pages of this book. But you do have to recognize that you have to make some permanent adjustments in your lifestyle for long-lasting success.

### *OPTIONAL*

It's your choice. This is not a dictatorial program. It's a benevolent, nonjudgmental system in which the weight loss and weight maintenance programs can be adapted to suit everyone's individual needs. You can use the Micro meals as your sole source of nutrition for faster weight loss, or take a more leisurely, modified approach.

### *SAFE*

Thousands of dieters have now been monitored in clinical trials involving nutritionally complete, very low-calorie and low-calorie diets. At least four million people worldwide have safely used The Micro Diet. It's a track record which speaks for itself.

### *EASY*

It's a simple, convenient program which anyone can follow. No calories to count. No foods to weigh. No portions to control. It really does take the guesswork out of dieting so that you don't "slip" and add unwanted, unnecessary calories. The meals are all prepared for you so you don't have to waste hours in the kitchen.

### *RAPID*

There is no faster, yet safe, way to lose your excess pounds—an average of fourteen pounds a month, consistently month-after-month, when following the 800-calorie-a-day plan. The only quicker way to lose weight would be by starving yourself.

### *FILLING*

Loser-Friendly dieters report that they find The Micro Diet to be completely satisfying. There are far fewer complaints of hunger when enjoying nutritionally complete meals as part of a low-calorie diet plan.

## *REALISTIC*

It's a very doable program. Based on sound recommendations from the U.S. *Surgeon General's Report,* The Micro Diet does not set you up to fail by making rash promises and giving you undue expectations. It is not a magic fix to the problem of being overweight. If you work with the program, it will work for you.

## *INTEGRITY*

You can be assured of the integrity of the Micro Diet products—the nutritional soundness and quality control—and you can be assured of the integrity of the people behind the program who have spent a decade advocating better health and nutrition through The Micro Diet.

## *ECONOMICAL*

The Micro Diet wins hands-down when compared with any other full-spectrum nutritionally complete weight-control system. Unlike some of the leading advertised programs there are no upfront fees or hidden costs.

## *NUTRITIOUS*

Three servings provide at least 100% of the U.S. government's Recommended Dietary Allowances of all essential micronutrients. Complete and balanced. No unnecessary megadoses. You also receive an excellent balance of the required amounts of protein, carbohydrate, and the essential fatty acids.

## *DELICIOUS*

The Micro Diet tastes great. Each meal has been created to appeal to the most discerning palate on the premise that dieters should enjoy meals and not be hoodwinked into thinking that meals have to be bland or medicinal "for their own good."

## *LIFE-CHANGING*

"It has changed my life." That's probably the most frequent comment I hear about The Micro Diet. No wonder. A whole new world is opened up for people who have shed their excess weight. They discover the joy of living. They report much more energy and an increased feeling of self-worth.

## *YOU'RE NEVER ALONE*

You can do it! It's all about you. It all comes down to you. You owe it to yourself to implement everything that you've learned. And by your side to help you every inch of the way will be the Micro Diet Advisor assigned to you. This flexible support system—tailored to your needs—is one of the great strengths of the program.

So have you just read this book or have you started to take action to produce results? Loser-Friendly, of course, is a play on the word User-Friendly which was introduced into the language with the advent of modern computer technology. But it's an ideal word to explain The Micro Diet program. It is user-friendly—with the emphasis on "friendly." The bond of friendship which is forged between the Micro Diet Advisor and the dieter can be the relationship that makes all the difference between success or failure.

The Loser-Friendly program, in my opinion, is the most realistic weight control system ever developed, giving you the freedom to eat that you've never had before because you can use Micro meals once or twice a day, or "sole source" for a day or two whenever necessary. If you don't regain more than a couple of pounds, you can't regain ten or twenty pounds. Don't allow more than a few pounds to creep back on your frame without taking action. It is vital, though, to act on the other dietary advice I have assembled for you in this book and make sure you obtain The Micro Diet's *Choices* program.

Here is a checklist of things you need to do. Use it and check each activity you complete each day. You may not need to do them all, but you will actually see just how much of the advice you are putting into practice. Please don't think, "That's a good idea," and run off to McDonald's. Do it.

You will not do everything at once. That's the mistake of old-style dieting. You can safely leave the weight-loss part to The Micro Diet. The checklist will get you thinking slim and acting slim permanently. Check off what you did. Then make a new checklist for next week. You'll soon see the gaps and so you'll automatically focus on doing these things next week.

No matter how many times you have tried to lose weight before, this time you can do it and, more importantly, keep it off. And remember, you're not alone. The entire Micro Diet family, the company, our Advisors, and our successful dieters coast-to-coast are with you every inch of the way. We want you to succeed just as much as you do, and we'll do everything we can to provide you with the support that you deserve.

## *THE MICRO DIET'S "STAY SLIM" CHECKLIST*

DID YOU:

- Keep a full record of what you ate (starting with a five-day commitment)?
- Eat at least three moderate-size meals, so you didn't become overly hungry?
- Eat slowly, chew thoroughly, and concentrate on the taste of the food?
- Eat only what you really wanted?
- Stop and become aware of how full you felt during the meal. Did you listen to your body?
- Stop eating when you were no longer hungry?
- Consciously leave something on your plate? Eat at planned meal times only, and only if you were hungry?
- Eat sitting down? Eat in the kitchen/dining room? Stop and ask yourself, "I can have it if I want it, but do I really want it?"
- Use The Micro Diet at least once a day. For breakfast? Lunch? Dinner?
- Do some brisk exercise of at least twenty minutes?
- React to negative feelings, e.g., boredom, tension, or upset by doing something active instead of eating?
- Consciously keep leftovers and "mindless" calories well out of sight?

- Tell a friend or Micro Diet Advisor about your progress?
- Do some "calorie trading" when you consciously decided you *really* did want an "extra"?
- Read the Easy Changes section of the book and make some of those substitutions?
- Remember that a binge is only a temporary reverse in your progress, so you need not worry unduly?
- Reduce or eliminate the "mindless calories"?
- Deliberately cut down on sugar and fat?
- Plan ahead how to deal with a future social situation?

## *MAKING A COMMITMENT*

You've been interested enough to read this far. That alone gives you an excellent chance of success. You are certain to succeed in losing weight with The Loser-Friendly Diet as long as you follow the directions. But keeping the weight off does definitely require some changes. These changes will be much easier because you now understand your body and your attitudes toward eating better.

Clearly, the more strongly motivated you are, the higher your chances of success. Answer "yes" to the following questions, sign where indicated, and get started.

I now realize that being overweight is a result of my eating too much for the way my body copes with food.

Yes/No

I know that to be significantly overweight brings health problems as you grow older. I won't let that happen to me.

Yes/No

I am too overweight for my own good, and I know it is jeopardizing my health.

Yes/No

I am prepared to use the "Stay Slim" Checklist for four weeks.

Yes/No

The person I care most about wants me to lose weight.

Yes/No

I really do see now that staying slim is a question of making a number of individually quite minor changes, but the accumulative effect is really worthwhile.

Yes/No

I am going to devote time to myself. I appreciate that getting and staying slim can be enjoyable.

Yes/No

I understand what's meant by "mindless calories" and am prepared to change the habit of consuming them.

Yes/No

I understand now that I sometimes eat, not just because I'm hungry, but for all sorts of other reasons. Now that I know that, I am prepared to react in a different way.

Yes/No

I am NOT just giving it a try, I am making a serious effort.

Yes/No

I know it will work, if I work with it.

Yes/No

________________________________

Your signature

________________________________

Your present weight

________________________________

Your goal weight

________________________________

Today's date

# HOW TO GET STARTED

You can become a Loser-Friendly success story. Join the winning dieters featured in this book by calling 1-800-934-TRIM or by taking advantage of the special introductory offer contained on the book flap. Send the coupon to Book Offer, Uni-Vite Inc., 2440 Impala Drive, Carlsbad, CA 92008.

You will be assigned your personal Micro Diet Advisor who will give you as much (or as little) support and encouragement as you want—free of charge. All that you will pay for are the healthy low-fat, low-calorie, meals which you will obtain directly from the Advisor. These delicious, nutritionally-complete meals are all under $3.00 each and are excellent quick-fix meals for the entire family.

# BIBLIOGRAPHY

Amatruda, J.M., et al. "Vigorous supplementation of a hypocaloric diet prevents cardiac arrythmias and mineral depletion." *American Journal of Medicine.* 1983. 1016-22.

Anderson, James W., et al. "Weight loss and 2-y follow-up for 80 morbidly obese patients treated with intensive very-low-calorie diet and education program." *Americal Journal of Clinical Nutrition.* 1992. 244S-6S.

Anderson, James W., et al. "Safety and effectiveness of a multidisciplinary very-low-calorie diet program for selected obese individuals." *Journal of the American Dietetic Association.* December 1991. 1582-4.

Anderson, James W., et al. "Results of a very-low-calorie diet/ behavioral weight loss program." *International Journal of Obesity.* 11. 4. 425A.

Apfelbaum, M., et al. "Effects of a high protein very-low-energy diet on ambulatory subjects with special reference to nitrogen balance." *International Journal of Obesity.* 1981. 117-30.

Apfelbaum, M., et al. "Low-and very-low-calorie diets." *American Journal of Clinical Nutrition.* 1987. 1126-34.

Arai, Keiko, et al. "Comparison of clinical usefulness of very-low-calorie diet and supplemental low-calorie diet." *American Journal of Clinical Nutrition.* 1992. 275S-6S.

Astrup, Arne, et al. "Dietary fibre added to very low calorie diet reduces hunger and alleviates constipation." *International Journal of Obesity.* 1990. 105-112.

Atkinson, Richard L., et al. "Combination of very-low-calorie diet and behavior modification in the treatment of obesity." *American Journal of Clinical Nutrition.* 1992. 199S-202S.

Atkinson, Richard L. "Low and very low calorie diets." *Medical Clinics of North America.* January 1989. 203-15.

Atkinson, Richard L. "Massive obesity: complications and treatment." *Nutrition Reviews.* February 1991. 49-53.

Ballor, Douglas L., et al. "Exercise intensity does not affect the composition of diet- and exercise-induced body mass loss." *American Journal of Clinical Nutrition.* 1990. 142-6.

Barrows, K., and J.T. Snook. "Effect of a high-protein, very-low-calorie diet on resting metabolism, thyroid hormones and energy expenditure of obese middle-aged women." *American Journal of Clinical Nutrition.* 1987. 391-8.

Beeson, V., et al. "The myth of the yo-yo; consistent rate of weight loss with successive dieting by VLCD." *International Journal of Obesity.* 1989. 13 (suppl 2.), 135-9.

Benotti, Peter N., et al. "Heart disease and hypertension in severe obesity: the benefits of weight reduction." *American Journal of Clinical Nutrition.* 1992. 586S-90S.

Bjorntorp, P. "The prevalence of obesity complications related to the distribution of surplus fat." *In Body Weight Control.* eds. Bender, A.E., and Brookes, L.J. Churchill Livingston. 1987.

Blackburn, G.L., and I. Greenburg. "Multidisciplinary approach to adult obesity therapy." *International Journal of Obesity.* 1978. 133-42.

Blackburn, G.L., et al. "Weight cycling; the experience of human dieters." *American Journal of Clinical Nutrition*. 1989. 1105-9.

Bloom, Walter Lyon. "Inhibition of salt excretion by carbohydrate." *Archives of Internal Medicine*. January 1962. 80-6.

Bloom, Walter Lyon, and William Mitchell Jr. "Salt excretion of fasting patients." *Archives of Internal Medicine*. September 1960. 321-26.

Bogardus, C., et al. "Metabolic fuels and the capacity for exercise during low calorie diets with or without carbohydrate." *Journal of Clinical Investigation*. 1981. 399-404.

Bolinger, Robert E., et al. "Metabolic balance of obese subjects during fasting." *Archives of Internal Medicine*. July 1966. 3-8.

Brownell, K.D., and R.W. Jeffrey. "Improving long-term weight loss: pushing the limits of treatment." *Behavior Therapy*. 1987. 353-74.

Burgess, Nancy Stearns. "Effect of a very-low-calorie diet on body composition and resting metabolic rate in obese men and women." *Research*. April 1991. 430-34.

Calles-Escandon, Jorge, and Edward S. Horton. "The thermogenic role of exercise in the treatment of morbid obesity: a critical evaluation." *American Journal of Clinical Nutrition*. 1992. 533S-7S.

Caviezel, F., et al. "Early improvement of left ventricular function during caloric restriction in obesity." *International Journal of Obesity*. 1986. 421-6.

Colditz, Graham A. "Economic costs of obesity." *American Journal of Clinical Nutrition*. 1992. 503S-7S.

Cox, Jacqueline S., et al. "Long-term outcome of a self-help very-low-calorie-diet weight-loss program." *American Journal of Clinical Nutrition*. 1992. 279S-80S.

Cummens, M.L. "Long term follow-up of obesity treated with very low calorie diet and intensive group psychotherapy." *International Journal of Obesity*. 1987. 11. 4. 449A.

Dale, D. van, and W. Saris. "Repetitive weight loss and weight regain: effects on weight reduction, resting metabolic rate, and lipolytic activity before and after exercise and/or diet treatment." *American Journal of Clinical Nutrition*. 1989. 409-16.

Davies, H.J.A., et al. "Metabolic response to low and very low calorie diets." *American Journal of Clinical Nutrition*. 1989. 745-51.

de Graaf, Cees, et al. "Short-term effects of different amounts of protein, fats, and carbohydrates on satiety." *American Journal of Clinical Nutrition*. 1992. 33-8.

Deitschuneit, H., et al. "Clinical experience with a very low calorie diet." *Management of Obesity by Severe Caloric Restriction*. PSG Publishing Co. 1985. 319-33.

Doherty, John U., et al. "Long-term evaluation of cardiac function in obese patients treated with a very-low-calorie diet: a controlled clinical study of patients without underlying cardiac disease." *American Journal of Clinical Nutrition*. 1991. 854-8.

Donnelly, Joseph E., et al. "Effects of a very-low-calorie diet and physical training regimens on body composition and resting metabolic rate in obese females." *American Journal of Clinical Nutrition*. 1991. 56-61.

Drenick, Ernst J., et al. "Prolonged starvation as treatment for severe obesity." *Journal of the American Medical Association*. January 11, 1964. 100-5.

Fisler, Janis S., and Ernst J. Drenick. "Starvation and semistarvation diets in the management of obesity." *Annual Review of Nutrition*. 1987. 465-84.

Fitzwater, Susan L., et al. "Evaluation of long-term weight changes after a multidisciplinary weight control program." *Journal of the American Dietetic Association*. April 1991. 421-29.

Forbes, G.B. "Do the obese gain weight more easily than the non-obese?" *International Journal of Obesity*. 1987. 11. 4. 425A.

Foreyt, John P., et al. "Limitations of behavorial treatment of obesity: review and analysis." *Journal of Behavioral Medicine*. 1981. 159-73.

Foster, Gary D., et al. "A controlled comparison of three very-low-calorie diets: effects on weight, body composition, and symptoms." *American Journal of Clinical Nutrition*. 1992. 811-7.

Foster, Gary D., et al. "Controlled trial of the metabolic effects of a very-low-calorie diet: short- and long-term effects." *American Journal of Clinical Nutrition*. 1990. 167-72.

Fricker, Jacques, et al. "Energy-metabolism adaptation in obese adults on a very-low-calorie diet." *American Journal of Clinical Nutrition*. 1991. 826-30.

Garrow, J.S. "Are liquid diets safe or necessary?" *Recent Advances in Obesity Research*. V. Berry, Blondheim, Eliahou and Shafrir (eds). John Libbey. 1987. 327-31.

Garrow, J.S., and Joan D. Webster. "Effects on weight and metabolic rate of obese women on a 3.4 (800 kcal) diet." *The Lancet*. June 24, 1989. 1429-31.

Gelfand, Robert A., and Rosa Hendler. "Effect of nutrient composition on the metabolic response to very low calorie diets: learning more and more about less and less." *Diabetes/Metabolism Reviews*. 1989. 17-30.

Genuth, S.M., et al. "Supplemented fasting in the treatment of obesity." *Recent Advances in Obesity Research II. ed. Bray, G.A. 1978. 370-8. Newman, London.*

Genuth, S.M. "Supplemented fasting in the treatment of obesity and diabetes." *American Journal of Clinical Nutrition.* 1979. 2579-86.

Goodrick, G. Kenneth, and John P. Foreyt. "Why treatments for obesity don't last." *Journal of the American Dietetic Association.* October 1991. 1243-47.

Hainer, Vojtech, et al. "Body-fat distribution and serum lipids during the long-term follow-up of obese patients treated initially with a very-low-calorie diet." *American Journal of Clinical Nutrition.* 1992. 283S-5S.

Halmi, Katherine A., et al. "Emotional responses to weight reduction by three methods: gastric bypass, jejunoileal bypass, diet." *American Journal of Clinical Nutrition.* February 1980. 446-51.

Hammer, R.L., et al. "Calorie-restricted low-fat diet and exercise in obese women." *American Journal of Clinical Nutrition.* 1989. 77-85.

Hendler, Rosa, and Alfons A. Bonde. "Very-low-calorie diets with high and low protein content: impact on triiodothyronine, energy expenditure, and nitrogen balance." *American Journal of Clinical Nutrition.* 1988. 1239-47.

Hendler, Rosa, and Alfons A. Bonde. "Effects of sucrose on resting metabolic rate, nitrogen balance, leucine turnover and oxidation during weight loss with low calorie diets." *International Journal of Obesity.* 1990. 927-938.

Henry, R.R., et al. "Glycemic effects of short-term intensive dietary restriction and isocaloric refeeding in non-insulin dependent diabetes mellitus." *Journal of Clinical Endocrinology and Metabolism.* 1986. 917-25.

Henry, R.R., et al. "Effects of weight loss on mechanisms of hyperglycemia in obese non-insulin-dependent diabetes mellitus." *Journal of the American Diabetes Association.* 1986. 9. 990-8.

Henry, R.R., et al. "Metabolic consequences of very low calorie diet therapy in obese non-insulin dependent diabetic and non-diabetic subjects." *Journal of the American Diabetes Association*. 1986. 155-64.

Hermann-Nickell, D., and T. Baker. "A multifactorial weight control program in a corporate setting." *Journal of the American Dietetic Association*. 1989. 534-7.

Heshka, Stanley, et al. "Weight loss and change in resting metabolic rate." *American Journal of Clinical Nutrition*. 1990. 981-6.

Hill, J.O., et al. "Effects of exercise and food restriction on body composition and metabolic rate in obese women." *American Journal of Clinical Nutrition*. 46. 622-630.

Hoffer, L.J., et al. "Metabolic effects of very low calorie weight reduction diets." *Journal of Clinical Investigation*. 1984.

Holmes, Michelle D., et al. "An analytic review of current therapies for obesity." *The Journal of Family Practice*. 1989. 610-16.

Hovell, Melbourne F., et al. "Long-term weight loss maintenance: assessment of a behavioral and supplemented fasting regimen." *American Journal of Public Health*. June 1988. 663-6.

Howard, A.N. "The historical development of very low calorie diets." *International Journal of Obesity*. 1989. 13 (suppl. 2).

Howard, A.N., et al. "The treatment of obesity with a very-low-calorie liquid-formula diet: an inpatient/outpatient comparison using skimmed milk protein as the chief protein source." *International Journal of Obesity*. 1978. 321-32.

Isner, J.M., et al. "Sudden unexpected death in avid dieters using the liquid protein-modified-fast diet. Observations in patients and the role of the prolonged QT interval." *Circulation*. 1979. 1401-12.

James, W.P.T. "Treatment of obesity: the constraints on success." *Clinics in Endocrinology and Metabolism.* 1984. 13.

Jebb, Susan A., et al. "Effects of weight cycling caused by intermittent dieting on metabolic rate and body composition in obese women." *International Journal of Obesity.* 1991. 367-74.

Jeffery, Robert W., et al. "Weight cycling and cardiovascular risk factors in obese men and women." *American Journal of Clinical Nutrition.* 1992. 641-4.

Johnston, Francis E., et al. "Body fat deposition in adult obese women. Patterns of fat distribution." *American Journal of Clinical Nutrition.* 1988. 225-8.

Jones, Jeffrey G. "Use of very-low-calorie diets in obesity." *American Family Physician.* volume 42, number 5.

Kamrath, Richard O., et al. "Body composition and weight maintenance with a very-low-calorie diet for the treatment of moderate obesity." *American Journal of Clinical Nutrition.* 1992. 286S-7S.

Kamrath, Richard O., et al. "Repeated use of the very-low-calorie diet in a structured multidisciplinary weight-management program." *American Journal of Clinical Nutrition.* 1992. 288S-9S.

Kanders, B.S., et al. "Weight loss outcome and health benefits associated with the Optifast program in the treatment of obesity." *International Journal of Obesity.* 13 (suppl. 2). 131-4.

Kaplan, Gordon D., et al. "Comparative weight loss in obese patients restarting a supplemented very-low-calorie diet." *American Journal of Clinical Nutrition.* 1992. 290S-1S.

Kirschner, M.A., et al. "An eight-year experience with a very-low-calorie formula diet for control of major obesity." *International Journal of Obesity.* 1988. 69-80.

Klesges, Robert C., et al. "The effects of smoking cessation and gender on dietary intake, physical activity, and weight gain." *International Journal of Eating Disorders.* 1990. 435-45.

Krotkiewski, Marcin, et al. "Increased muscle dynamic endurance associated with weight reduction on very-low-calorie diet." *American Journal of Clinical Nutrition.* 1990. 321-30.

Kuczmarski, Robert J. "Prevalence of overweight and weight gain in the United States." *American Journal of Clinical Nutrition.* 1992. 495S-502S.

Lantigua, R.A., et al. "Cardiac arrhythmias associated with a liquid protein diet for the treatment of obesity." *New England Journal of Medicine.* 1980. 735-8.

Laporte, David J., and Albert J. Stunkard. "Predicting attrition and adherence to a very low calorie diet: a prospective investigation of the eating inventory." *International Journal of Obesity.* 1990. 197-206.

Larsson, Bo. "Obesity, fat distribution and cardiovascular disease." *International Journal of Obesity.* 1991. 53-7.

Lemons, A.D., et al. *International Journal of Obesity.* 13 (suppl. 2) 119-23.

Lissner, Lauren, et al. "Variability of body weight and health outcomes in the Framingham population." *New England Journal of Medicine.* 1991. 1839-44.

MacMahon, S.W., et al. "The effect of weight reduction on left ventricular mass. A randomized controlled trial in young, overweight hypertensive patients." *New England Journal of Medicine.* 1986. 334-9.

Manson, J.E., et al. "A prospective study of obesity and risk of coronary heart disease in women." *New England Journal of Medicine.* 1990. 322.

Millar, Wayne J., and Thomas Stephens. "The prevalence of overweight and obesity in Britain, Canada, and United States." *American Journal of Public Health.* January 1987. 38-41.

Moyer, C.L., et al. "Effects of cardiac stress during a very low calorie diet and exercise program in obese women." *American Journal of Clinical Nutrition.* 1989. 1324-7.

National Academy of Sciences -- National Research Council, Recommended Dietary Allowances. Revised 1980. Food and Nutrition Board.

National Institutes of Health. "Technology assessment conference statement: methods for voluntary weight loss and control." April 1, 1992. 1-36.

Olefsky, J.M. *Diabetes Mellitus.* In 17th Edition, Cecil text book. J.B. Wyngaardenand and L.H. Smith (eds). W.B. Saunders Company. 1984. 1320-43.

Pavlou, K.N., et al. "Effects of dieting and exercise on lean body mass, oxygen uptake and strength." *Medicine and Science in Sports and Exercise.* 1985. 17. 4. 466-71.

Phinney, Stephen D. "Exercise during and after very-low-calorie dieting." *American Journal of Clinical Nutrition.* 1992. 109S-14S.

Phinney, S.D., et al. "Capacity for moderate exercise in obese subjects after adaptation to a hypocaloric, ketogenic diet." *Journal of Clinical Investigation.* 1980. 1152-61.

Pi-Sunyer, F. Xavier. "Health implications of obesity." *American Journal of Clinical Nutrition.* 1991. 1595S-1603S.

Prentice, Andrew M., et al. "Effects of weight cycling on body composition." *American Journal of Clinical Nutrition.* 1992. 209S-16S.

Rand, Colleen S.W., and Alex M.C. Macgregor. "Successful weight loss following obesity surgery and the perceived liability of morbid obesity." *International Journal of Obesity*. 1991. 577-79.

Rimm, Alfred A., et al. "Relationship of obesity and disease in 73,532 weight-conscious women." *Public Health Reports*. January-February 1975. 44-51.

Rolls, Barbara J. "Effects of intense sweeteners on hunger, food intake, and body weight: a review." *American Journal of Clinical Nutrition*. 1991. 872-8.

Safer, Daniel J. "Diet, behavior modification, and exercise: a review of obesity treatments from a long-term perspective." *Southern Medical Journal*. December 1991. 1470-74.

Saris, Wim H.M., et al. "Outcome of a multicenter outpatient weight-management program including very-low-calorie diet and exercise." *American Journal of Clinical Nutrition*. 1992. 294S-6S.

Schouten, J.A., et al. "The influence of low calorie (240 kcal/day) protein-carbohydrate diet on serum lipid levels in obese subjects." *International Journal of Obesity*. 1981. 333-9.

Sikand, Geeta, et al. "Two-year follow-up of patients treated with a very-low-calorie diet and exercise training." *Journal of the American Dietetic Association*. April 1988. 487-8.

Sours, H.E., et al. "Sudden death associated with very low calorie weight reduction regimens." *American Journal of Clinical Nutrition*. 34. 453-61.

Spencer, I.O.B., and M.B. Durh. "Death during therapeutic starvation for obesity." *The Lancet*. June 15, 1968. 1288-90.

Stern, J.S., et al. "Obesity: does exercise make a difference?" *Recent Advances in Obesity Research*. V. John Libbey & Co., London. 1987.

Stevens, V., et al. "Freedom from fat: a contemporary multicomponent weight loss program for the general population of obese adults." *Journal of the American Dietetic Association*. 1989. 1254-8.

Striegel-Moore, Ruth, et al. "Psychological and behavorial correlates of feeling fat in women." *International Journal of Eating Disorders*. 1986. 935-47.

Stunkard, Albert J., and H.C. Berthold. "What is behavior therapy? A very short description of behavior weight control." *American Journal of Clinical Nutrition*. 821-3.

Stunkard, Albert J., et al. "An adoption study of human obesity." *New England Journal of Medicine*. 1986 193-8.

Stunkard, Albert J., and Thomas A. Wadden. "Psychological aspects of severe obesity." *American Journal of Clinical Nutrition*. 1992. 524S-32S.

*The Surgeon General's Report on Nutrition and Health*. U.S. Department of Health and Human Services, 1988.

Suter, Paolo M., et al. "The effect of ethanol on fat storage in healthy subjects." *New England Journal of Medicine*. 1992. 983-7.

Tuck, M.L., et al. "The effect of weight reduction on blood pressure, plasma renin activity and plasma aldosterone levels in obese patients." *New England Journal of Medicine*. 1981, 930-3.

Tufts University Diet & Nutrition Letter. Vol. 6: No. 12.

Uusitupa, Matti I.J., et al. "Effects of a very-low-calorie diet on metabolic control and cardiovascular risk factors in the treatment of obese non-insulin-dependent diabetics." *American Journal of Clinical Nutrition*. 1990. 768-73.

Van Dale, D., and W.M.H. Saris. "Repetitive weight loss and regain; effects on weight reduction, resting metabolic rate and lipolytic activity before and after exercise and/or diet treatment." *American Journal of Clinical Nutrition*. 1989. 49.

Van Gaal, L.F., et al. "Anthropometric and calorimetric evidence for the protein sparing effects of a new protein supplemented low calorie preparation." *American Journal of Clinical Nutrition.* 1985. 41.

Van Itallie, T.B. "Health implications of overweight and obesity in the United States, National Institutes of Health Consensus Development Conference." *Annals of Internal Medicine.* 1985. 103. 6. 1073-7.

Vertes, V. "Very low calorie diets—history, safety and recent developments." *Postgraduate Medical Journal.* 1984. 56-8.

Vertes, V., et al. "Supplemented fasting as a large-scale out-patient program." *Journal of the American Medical Association.* 1977. 238 (20). 2151-3.

Wadden, Thomas A., and A.J. Stunkard. "Controlled trial of very low calorie diet, behavior therapy and their combination in the treatment of obesity." *Journal of Consulting and Clinical Psychology.* 1986. 4. 482-8.

Wadden, Thomas A., et al. "Relationships of dieting history to resting metabolic rate, body composition, eating behavior, and subsequent weight loss." *American Journal of Clinical Nutrition.* 1992. 203S-8S.

Wadden, Thomas A., et al. "Clinical correlates of short- and long-term weight loss." *American Journal of Clinical Nutrition.* 1992. 271S-4S.

Wadden, Thomas A., et al. "A comparison of two very low calorie diets: protein sparing modified fast versus protein formula liquid diet." *American Journal of Clinical Nutrition.* 1985. 533-9.

Wadden, Thomas A., et al. "Very low calorie diets: their efficacy, safety and future." *Annals of Internal Medicine.* 1983. 675-84.

Wadden, Thomas A., et al. "Less food, less hunger: reports of appetite and symptoms in a controlled study of a protein-sparing modified fast." *International Journal of Obesity.* 1987. 239-49.

Wadden, Thomas A., et al. "Three-year follow-up of the treatment of obesity by very low calorie diet, behavior therapy, and their combination." *Journal of Consulting and Clinical Psychology*. 1988. 925-8.

Wadden, Thomas A., et al. "Effects of a very low calorie diet on weight, thyroid hormones and mood." *International Journal of Obesity*. 1990. 249-58.

Wadden, Thomas A., et al. "Responsible and irresponsible use of very-low-calorie diets in the treatment of obesity." *Journal of the American Medical Association*. 1990. 83-5.

Webster, J.D., and J.S. Garrow. "Weight loss in 108 obese women on a diet supplying 800 kcal/d for 21 d." *American Journal of Clinical Nutrition*. 1989. 41-5.

Williamson, David F., et al. "The 10-year incidence of overweight and major weight gain in U.S. adults." *Archives of Internal Medicine*. 1990. 665-72.

Wilson, J.H.P., and S.W.J. Lamberts. "Nitrogen balance in obese patients receiving a very low calorie liquid formula diet." *American Journal of Clinical Nutrition*. 1979. 32.

Wing, Rena R., and R.W. Jeffrey. "Outpatient treatments of obesity: a comparison of methodology and clinical results." *International Journal of Obesity*. 3. 261-72.

Wing, Rena R. "Don't throw out the baby with the bathwater. A commentary on very-low-calorie diets." *Diabetes Care*. 1992. 293-96.

Wing, Rena R., et al. "Psychological responses of obese type II diabetic subjects to very-low-calorie diet." *Diabetes Care*. 1991. 596-99.

Wooley, Susan C., and David M. Garner. "Obesity treatment: the high cost of false hope." *Journal of the American Dietetic Association*. 1991. 1248-51.

Wynn, V., et al. "Method of estimating rate of fat loss during treatment of obesity by calorie restriction." *The Lancet*. 1985. 482-6.

Yang, M.U., et al. "Metabolic effects of substituting carbohydrate for protein in a low calorie diet; a prolonged study in obese patients." *International Journal of Obesity*. 1981. 231-6.

Zorbas, Yan G., et al. "Effect of low-calorie diets on metabolism of man under hypokinesia." *JEPTO*. 457-65.

# INDEX